The Endocrine System

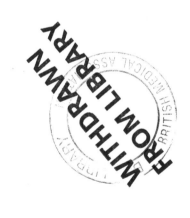

This book is dedicated to the memory of Dr Saad Al-Damluji, endocrinologist and teacher

Commissioning Editor: Timothy Horne
Development Editor: Lulu Stader
Project Manager: Janaki Srinivasan Kumar
Designer/Design Direction: Charles Gray
Illustration Manager: Gillian Richards

SYSTEMS OF THE BODY

The Endocrine System

BASIC SCIENCE AND CLINICAL CONDITIONS

SECOND EDITION

JOY HINSON   BSc PhD DSc FHEA
Professor of Endocrine Science
Dean for Postgraduate Studies
Barts and the London School of Medicine and Dentistry
Queen Mary University of London
London, UK

PETER RAVEN   BSc PhD MBBS MRCP MRCPsych FHEA
Faculty Tutor (Biomedical Sciences), UCL
Deputy Director of Medical Education, UCL Medical School
and Honorary Consultant Psychiatrist
Camden and Islington Mental Health Trust
London, UK

SHERN CHEW   BSc MD FRCP
Professor of Endocrine Medicine/Consultant Physician
Barts and the London School of Medicine and Dentistry
Queen Mary University of London
London, UK

Illustrations by Robert Britton

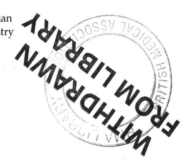

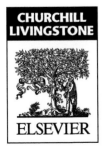

CHURCHILL LIVINGSTONE

ELSEVIER

EDINBURGH LONDON NEW YORK OXFORD PHILADELPHIA ST LOUIS SYDNEY TORONTO 2010

CHURCHILL
LIVINGSTONE
ELSEVIER

First Edition Elsevier Limited, 2007.
Second Edition © 2010, Elsevier Limited. All rights reserved.
Reprinted in 2012, 2013, 2014 (twice) and 2015

ISBN 978-0-7020-3372-8

British Library Cataloguing in Publication Data
A catalogue record for this book is available from the British Library

Library of Congress Cataloging in Publication Data
A catalog record for this book is available from the Library of Congress

Notice
Knowledge and best practice in this field are constantly changing. As new research and experience broaden our knowledge, changes in practice, treatment and drug therapy may become necessary or appropriate. Readers are advised to check the most current information provided (i) on procedures featured or (ii) by the manufacturer of each product to be administered, to verify the recommended dose or formula, the method and duration of administration, and contraindications. It is the responsibility of the practitioner, relying on their own experience and knowledge of the patient, to make diagnoses, to determine dosages and the best treatment for each individual patient, and to take all appropriate safety precautions. To the fullest extent of the law, neither the Publisher nor the Authors assume any liability for any injury and/or damage to persons or property arising out of or related to any use of the material contained in this book.

The Publisher

 your source for books, journals and multimedia in the health sciences

www.elsevierhealth.com

Printed in Great Britain

Endocrinology is really very simple. You can either have too much of a hormone … or too little.

(Professor John Landon's traditional and reassuring introduction to his endocrinology teaching.)

The first edition of this book was aimed primarily at medical students, particularly those taking a modern, integrated course. This second edition is enlarged and expanded to include more detail of physiological and biochemical mechanisms, and has a whole chapter on mechanisms of hormone action. We hope that this edition will be used by students of the biomedical sciences as well as medical students.

The book is intended as a broad general introduction to the Endocrine System, although we hope that you will be sufficiently enthused after reading it to wish to take your studies further in this exciting and fast-moving area.

Each chapter is structured around clinical cases. Endocrinology is at its most interesting when considered in the context of what happens when things go wrong. These cases have been chosen to illustrate important points about either the biochemistry of hormone synthesis or the physiology of endocrine regulation. This will allow medical students early in their studies to understand the clinical relevance of the basic science. However, we hope that the book will also allow clinical students to understand the basic science underlying endocrine disease.

In the clinical cases featured in this book we have tried to show common presentations of the different disorders, but endocrine problems present in such a wide variety of ways that students should not be misled into thinking that these are the only presentations!

The 'Interesting fact' we included in the first edition have been added to. These are snippets of information that particularly interested us and that we wanted to share with you. We hope that you will find them interesting too.

The first two chapters are not case-based: these contain details of the basic concepts needed to understand hormones and their actions. The final chapter describes a mixture of hormones and other signalling molecules with varying degrees of clinical importance. This chapter illustrates perfectly the idea that endocrinology is rather more than a stand-alone speciality but rather it is a subject which impinges on the cardiovascular system, the immune system and all other systems of the body.

We do hope that we have managed to convey to you our enthusiasm for this most fascinating subject.

ACKNOWLEDGEMENTS

We are most grateful to all our colleagues for their help and advice in the preparation of this book. In particular, we would like to thank: Dr Dan Berney for providing the histology, Dr Norbert Avril for the whole-body glucose image and Dr Alistair Chesser for the EPO case. Thanks also to Dr Antonia Brooke, Derek and Niloufar (you know why), Dr John Patterson and Mrs Jacqualyn Conner. Although many colleagues have helped and advised us, all errors remain our own.

Thanks are due also to the team at Elsevier led by Timothy Horne, and especially to our editor, Lulu Stader.

CONTENTS

CONTENTS

INTRODUCTION

1

Chapter objectives

After studying this chapter you should be able to:

1. Explain what is meant by a hormone and name the major endocrine organs.

2. Categorize common hormones by their basic chemical structures.

3. Understand the role of plasma binding proteins for some hormones.

4. Understand the different forms of endocrine regulation, including set point, diurnal variation, endocrine axis and negative feedback.

5. Understand the basis of endocrine disease.

6. Appreciate the purpose and types of endocrine testing.

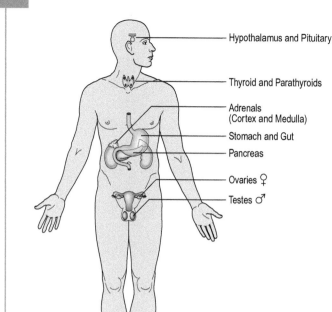

Figure 1.1 Major endocrine glands of the body. In addition, the gut, heart and skin have all been shown to produce hormones.

Hypothalamus and Pituitary

Thyroid and Parathyroids

Adrenals
(Cortex and Medulla)

Stomach and Gut

Pancreas

Ovaries ♀

Testes ♂

What is endocrinology?

Endocrinology is the study of hormones and their actions. Hormones are chemical messengers, released into the blood, that act through receptors to cause a change in the target cell. The glands that release hormones are ductless, giving the term 'endocrine' from the Greek for 'internal secretion'. The thyroid gland is an example of a classical endocrine gland. Its only function is to synthesize and release hormones into the bloodstream. Some organs, such as the pancreas, have endocrine as well as other functions. So the hormones released by the pancreas are released directly into the blood, whereas the other (exocrine) secretions of the pancreas are released into a duct.

The major, or 'classical', endocrine glands are shown in Figure 1.1 and the hormones they secrete are listed in Table 1.1. It has been suggested that the vascular endothelium, the whole gastrointestinal tract, and even the skin, should also be considered to be endocrine organs as they all release hormones or their precursors into the blood. Such tissues form the extensive 'diffuse endocrine system', which is located throughout the body. This system consists of scattered endocrine cells, located in various different tissues, that secrete hormones but do not form a discrete endocrine gland.

Endocrinology is a relatively young branch of medical science and is, by definition, exciting. The term

'hormone' was coined by Starling in the early 1900s. It derives from the Greek *hormon*, meaning 'exciting' or 'setting in motion'. Ernest Starling (1866–1927) is perhaps best known for his eponymous law of the cardiovascular system, but is also regarded as the founder of endocrinology. Working at University College, London, with Sir William Bayliss, he isolated and described the actions of secretin, the first known hormone. Starling built on the theoretical work of Edward Schafer and developed the concept of 'an endocrine system' in 1905, in a series of lectures called 'On the chemical correlations of the functions of the body'.

Endocrine disorders are very common in Western society and it has been estimated that more than half the population will suffer from an endocrine disease during their lifetime. There are several examples of common endocrine diseases: osteoporosis, the bone-weakening disease, affects one-third of older women. Around one in six women has polycystic ovarian disease. In addition, an increasing number of the population has type 2 diabetes, a disease of insulin resistance, as a result of obesity.

Interesting fact

The year 2005 saw the centenary of 'Endocrinology' as a recognized science and branch of medicine. Learned societies, such as the Society for Endocrinology, celebrated this with a series of special published articles, papers, lectures, events and poster campaigns (Fig. 1.2). To put this into perspective, surgery and pharmacology have been around for thousands of years.

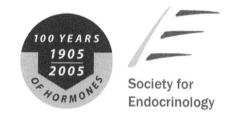

Society for Endocrinology

Figure 1.2 In 2005, The Society for Endocrinology celebrated the centenary of Endocrinology as a recognized science.

What do hormones do?

There are two major regulatory systems in the body: the neural system and the endocrine system. Although both use chemical messengers, they are set up very differently and have quite different functions. Neural regulation is very rapid, while endocrine control is generally slower and acts over a longer period of time. These differences arise because the neural system is designed to deliver its messenger directly to the surface of its target cell, while the endocrine system puts its messengers into the blood and allows for diffusion from the

Table 1.1 Major endocrine glands and the hormones they secrete

Gland	Hormone	Type of hormone
Hypothalamus	Corticotropin releasing hormone (CRH)	Peptide
	Dopamine (DA)	Modified amino acid
	Gonadotropin-releasing hormone (GnRH)	Peptide
	Growth hormone releasing hormone (GHRH)	Peptide
	Somatostatin	Peptide
	Thyrotropin-releasing hormone (TRH)	Peptide
	Vasopressin (AVP; anti-diuretic hormone, ADH)	Peptide
Anterior pituitary	Adrenocorticotropic (ACTH)	Peptide
	Follicle stimulating hormone (FSH)	Peptide
	Growth hormone (GH)	Peptide
	Luteinizing hormone (LH)	Peptide
	Prolactin (Prl)	Peptide
	Thyroid stimulating hormone (TSH; thyrotropin)	Peptide
Posterior pituitary	Oxytoxin	Peptide
	Vasopressin (AVP; anti-diuretic hormone, ADH)	Peptide
Thyroid	Thyroxine (T4)	Modified amino acid
	Tri-iodothyronine (T3)	Modified amino acid
	Calcitonin	Peptide
Parathyroid	Parathyroid hormone (PTH)	Peptide
Adrenal cortex	Aldosterone	Steroid
	Cortisol	Steroid
	Dehydroepiandrosterone (DHEA)	Steroid
Adrenal medulla	Adrenaline (epinephrine)	Modified amino acid
	Noradrenaline (norepinephrine)	Modified amino acid
Pancreas	Insulin	Peptide
	Glucagon	Peptide
Stomach and gut	Gastrin	Peptide
	Glucagon	Peptide
	Vasoactive intestinal polypeptide (VIP)	Peptide
	And many other peptides, see Ch. 13	
Ovaries	17 beta oestradiol	Steroid
	Progesterone	Steroid
Testes	Testosterone	Steroid
Kidneys	Erythropoietin (EPO)	Peptide
	Calcitriol	Modified steroid

blood to the target cell. Thus, the endocrine system is not designed for the same speed of communication as the neural system, but instead has the ability to deliver its messengers to a wider range of targets throughout the body.

Hormones usually control regulatory systems in the body, including homeostasis, metabolism and reproduction. Homeostasis means 'keeping the same' and is a term used to describe the regulation of any of the large physiological systems in the body, including levels of glucose in blood and body temperature. Hormones are particularly important in making sure that blood levels of sodium, potassium, calcium and glucose stay within set limits.

The boundaries between the endocrine system and the neural system are quite fuzzy (Fig. 1.3), because some hormones are released from nerve endings, 'neurohormones', while other hormones, such as adrenaline, are perhaps better known as neurotransmitters.

Types of hormone: their synthesis and secretion

In terms of their chemical structure, hormones are a varied group of substances. There are, however, three major basic types. The first and most numerous are the peptide hormones, made of chains of amino acids. Some of these are very small indeed: the hypothalamic hormone thyrotropin releasing hormone (TRH) is only three amino acids long, whereas the pituitary hormone whose release it stimulates (thyroid stimulating hormone, TSH) is a large glycoprotein with a molecular weight of around 30 000 Daltons. Usually, peptide hormones are pre-formed and stored in granules within the endocrine cell, ready for release in response to the appropriate signal. The synthesis and secretion of peptide hormones is shown in Figure 1.4A.

Many peptide hormones, particularly the larger ones, undergo modification of the basic peptide sequence before being secreted. This post-translational processing, which occurs in the Golgi apparatus and the secretory granules, can include the linking of peptide chains by disulphide bridges, and the addition of carbohydrate residues (glycosylation). Peptide hormone-secreting cells are distinguished by the large amounts of rough endoplasmic reticulum, prominent Golgi apparatus and by the presence of secretory granules, containing the finished hormone ready for secretion.

The second major group of hormones consists of the steroids. These are all made from cholesterol (Fig. 1.4B) and have a common core structure (Fig. 1.5). Quite small chemical changes to this core structure cause significant differences in their biological effects (Fig. 1.6). The steroids are formed by metabolism of cholesterol by enzymes within the steroid-secreting cell, located either within the mitochondria or the smooth endoplasmic reticulum. Cells which are involved in steroid hormone production are distinctive under microscopy because of the presence of unusually large amounts of smooth endoplasmic reticulum and mitochondria. They also usually contain significant lipid droplets, containing cholesterol esters, as steroid-secreting cells store the precursor to hormone synthesis rather than the finished product. The pathways of steroid hormone biosynthesis are shown in the adrenal chapter and the chapters on reproduction.

The third group of hormones are those derived from amino acids. For example, tyrosine residues can be iodinated to give thyroid hormones, or hydroxylated as the first step on the biosynthetic pathway of the

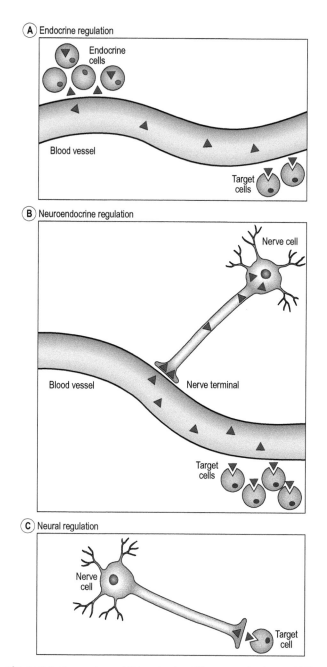

Figure 1.3 Comparison of (A) endocrine, (B) neuroendocrine and (C) neural regulation. In endocrine regulation, the hormone is released from the cells of an endocrine or 'ductless' gland into the bloodstream where the hormones travel to target cells often at some distance from the endocrine gland. In neural regulation, the neurotransmitter is released, in response to an action potential, from a nerve ending into the synaptic cleft, directly onto the surface of the target cell. In neuroendocrine regulation, the hormone is secreted by a nerve cell in response to an action potential, but is released into the bloodstream, not a synaptic cleft, and then acts as a hormone.

catecholamines: dopamine, adrenaline and noradrenaline (Fig. 1.7). A detailed account of the synthesis of thyroid hormones in given in Chapter 7 and for the catecholamines, in Chapter 5.

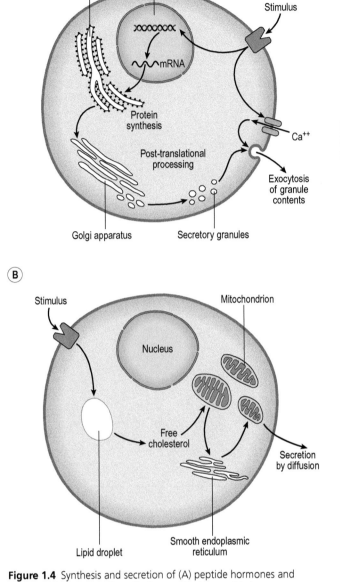

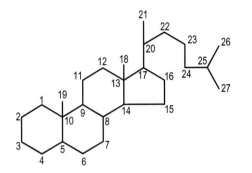

Figure 1.5 Structure of cholesterol, the parent compound for all steroid hormones and vitamin D. The classical steroid system for numbering carbon atoms is shown.

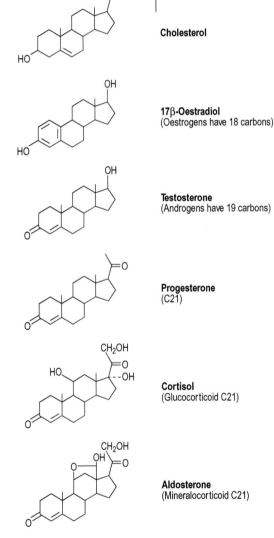

Figure 1.6 The major families of steroid hormones.

Figure 1.4 Synthesis and secretion of (A) peptide hormones and (B) steroid hormones. The cells that synthesize peptide hormones have abundant rough endoplasmic reticulum and Golgi apparatus. Secretory granules are often visible. Peptides require a specific secretory mechanism, exocytosis, which is usually triggered by an increase in intracellular calcium levels, or depolarization of the cell. The entire contents of the secretory granule are released. Steroid-secreting cells, on the other hand, have lipid droplets visible in the cytoplasm. They have abundant mitochondria and smooth endoplasmic reticulum. The steroid hormones, once made, simply diffuse out of the cell and do not require a specific secretory mechanism.

The differences in chemical structure of hormones have implications for the way in which these hormones are stored, released, transported in blood, their mechanism of action and, of course, their route of administration when they are used therapeutically (Table 1.2). Peptide hormones and catecholamines, being generally quite water-soluble, dissolve readily in plasma, the fluid component of the blood, but cannot enter the target cell, so interact with receptors on the cell surface. The lipophilic steroid and thyroid hormones, on the other hand, dissolve poorly in plasma and are mostly transported in blood bound to carrier proteins, but readily enter cells to interact with cytoplasmic or nuclear receptors. While peptide hormones and catecholamines are synthesized then stored in granules in the cells to be released as soon as they are needed (see Fig. 1.4A), steroid-secreting cells keep a store of cholesterol, the substrate for steroid biosynthesis, rather than the final steroid product (see Fig. 1.4B). This is largely a matter of practicality as the steroid hormones, being lipid soluble, are difficult to store, whereas cholesterol can be esterified and stored easily. Similarly, in the thyroid gland, a store of precursor is maintained, from which thyroid hormones may be readily released.

As a consequence of their small and lipophilic nature, steroid hormones do not require a specific secretory mechanism: they simply diffuse across the plasma membrane and out of the cell down a concentration gradient. Peptide hormones, on the other hand, need a specific secretory mechanism (see Fig. 1.4).

Finally, when they are used therapeutically, steroid hormones and thyroid hormones are orally active, whereas most peptide hormones (such as insulin) must be injected, to avoid being inactivated by digestive enzymes.

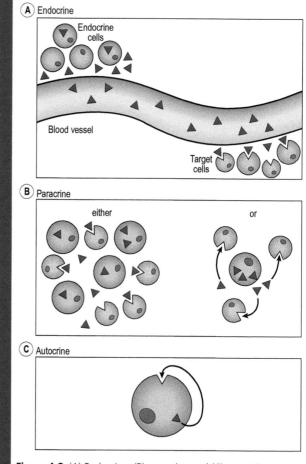

Figure 1.8 (A) Endocrine, (B) paracrine and (C) autocrine regulation.

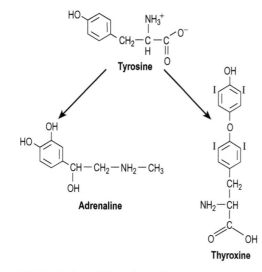

Figure 1.7 Metabolism of the amino acid tyrosine produces both thyroid hormones (thyroxine) and catecholamines (adrenaline).

Table 1.2 Comparison of steroids, peptides, thyroid hormones and catecholamines

	Location of receptors	Carrier protein	Active if administered orally?	Storage
Peptides	Cell membrane	No	Not usually	Hormone stored
Steroids	Cytoplasm/nucleus	Yes	Yes, mostly	Precursor stored
Thyroid hormone	Nucleus	Yes	Yes	Precursor stored
Catecholamines	Cell membrane	No	No	Hormone stored

The transport and metabolism of hormones

Hormones circulate in blood in very low concentrations indeed, and for this reason they are measured in units that are unfamiliar to many people (Table 1.3). Although some hormones, mostly the peptide hormones, are freely water-soluble, the steroid and thyroid hormones are not so soluble, and need to be transported in blood bound to a carrier or binding protein (Table 1.4). Not all steroids have a specific binding protein: aldosterone, for example, does not have a specific carrier protein, and circulates in blood mostly bound loosely to albumin. The binding proteins have three main functions. First, they increase the solubility of the hormone in blood. Second, they create a readily accessible reserve of the hormone in blood. Only the fraction of hormone that is not bound to the carrier protein is considered to be biologically active. When we describe a hormone as 'biologically active' we mean that it is available to exert its physiological effects but is also susceptible to metabolism or excretion. The biologically active hormone is 'seen' by the body but the bound hormone is effectively hidden. This is one factor that must be considered when measuring circulating concentrations of hormones: some assays measure total hormone (bound and free) while others measure only the biologically active hormone. You really need to know what it is that you are measuring. It is particularly important because levels of binding proteins can be altered in some clinical conditions and by some drugs.

The third function is to increase the biological half-life of the hormone. The biological half-life of a hormone is the time taken for half the hormone present in blood to be metabolized or excreted. It can be measured by injecting somebody with a 'tagged' hormone that can be easily distinguished from the normal hormone, then seeing how quickly it disappears from the circulation by measuring the amount present in samples taken at different times after the injection (Fig. 1.9). Binding proteins increase the biological half-life of a hormone by protecting it from metabolism and excretion, so that aldosterone, which does not have a specific carrier protein, has a half-life of around 15 min, whereas cortisol, which is bound to cortisol binding globulin (CBG), has a half-life of 90 min.

Different types of hormones are metabolized and excreted in different ways: Peptide hormones are mainly metabolized following binding to a receptor in the target cell. The hormone–receptor complex is internalized (that is taken up into the cell), and the hormone undergoes degradation in a lysosome. Most peptide hormones have a short half-life of just a few minutes, although the larger glycosylated peptide hormones such as thyroid stimulating hormone and luteinizing hormone have a longer half-life.

Steroid hormones are small and lipophilic and may be excreted by the kidney in an unchanged form. Mostly,

Table 1.4 Hormones and their binding proteins

Hormone	Binding protein
Thyroid hormone	Thyroid hormone binding globulin (THBG)
Testosterone/oestradiol	Sex hormone binding globulin (SHBG)
Cortisol	Cortisol binding globulin (CBG, also called transcortin)
Vitamin D	Vitamin D binding protein (DBP)

Table 1.3 Concentrations of various substances in blood

Substance	Concentration in SI units (using conventional abbreviations)	Log mol/L and equivalent SI unit (per litre) in full	
Sodium	140 mmol/L	10^{-1}	100 millimoles
Bicarbonate	21–26 mmol/L	10^{-2}	10 millimoles
Glucose	3–5 mmol/L	10^{-3}	1 millimole
Uric acid	150–500 µmol/L	10^{-4}	100 micromoles
Iron	10–30 µmol/L	10^{-5}	10 micromoles
Vitamin A	0.5–2 µmol/L	10^{-6}	1 micromole
Cortisol (0900 h)	200–650 nmol/L	10^{-7}	100 nanomoles
Testosterone (men)	10–35 nmol/L	10^{-8}	10 nanomoles
Tri-iodothyronine	1–3.5 nmol/L	10^{-9}	1 nanomole
Adrenaline (resting)	170–500 pmol/L	10^{-10}	100 picomoles
Free thyroxine	10–30 pmol/L	10^{-11}	10 picomoles
Oxytocin (basal)	1–4 pmol/L	10^{-12}	1 picomole

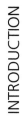

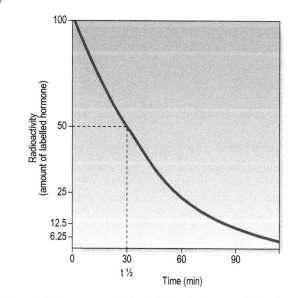

Figure 1.9 Measurement of the half-life of a hormone in blood. A labelled (radioactive) hormone is injected into the blood at time 0. Blood is sampled regularly and the radioactive content measured. When there is half the original level, the interval between time 0 and this time is called the half-life (t½) of the hormone. In the example shown, the plasma half-life of the hormone is 30 min.

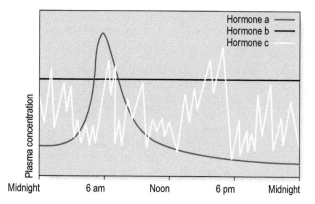

Figure 1.10 Diurnal variation and episodic secretion. Some hormones, such as hormone a, have a pronounced diurnal variation in their secretion. An example of such a hormone would be cortisol. Other hormones such as hormone b, which could be thyroxine, show very little diurnal variation. Hormone c shows episodic secretion; this pattern is common to many different hormones. It means that taking a single-point blood measurement of the hormone is of little value in diagnosing endocrine disorder because there is so much variation during the day.

however, they undergo metabolism in the liver into more water-soluble forms which are then excreted in bile and in the urine. Catecholamines are metabolized rapidly by the action of an enzyme called catechol-O-methyltransferase (COMT) which is found in most tissues but especially blood vessels, and by monoamine oxidase (MAO) in neural tissues.

Metabolism of hormones does not only result in their inactivation, however. There are examples of the principal secreted hormone being inactive and requiring metabolism in peripheral tissues to produce the active version. Testosterone is a good example of this: it needs to be metabolized to 5-alpha dihydrotestosterone in order to have its effects in its target tissues. Similarly, metabolism of Vitamin D3 is absolutely essential to produce the active calcitriol.

The metabolism of thyroxine is by the removal of one of the iodine residues of the hormone. Depending on which particular iodine residue is removed this either increases the activity of the hormone by producing T3, or decreases the activity by producing reverse T3. So we can see that metabolism, as well as providing a way of excreting hormones more efficiently, can also provide a way of regulating the activity of the hormone.

Important concepts in endocrine regulation

There are several concepts which are important for the understanding of endocrinology. These include the understanding of different patterns of hormone secretion,

the concept of an 'endocrine axis', the idea of negative feedback regulation, and the concepts of hormone antagonism and synergy.

Patterns of hormone secretion (Fig. 1.10)

Episodic secretion

The endocrine system is involved in a variety of homeostatic mechanisms in the body. In many cases regulation involves the maintenance of a 'set point' by correction of any deviation from this point. One example is the regulation of plasma calcium concentration, which is tightly controlled within closely set limits. In this case, any deviation from the set point triggers a hormonal response which acts to correct the calcium level (see Ch. 12). This results in the episodic secretion of the regulatory hormone. Other hormones are also secreted episodically, not because they are responding to physiological changes but because they are always secreted episodically or in bursts. These bursts can be quite frequent. For example, if you took very frequent blood samples to measure levels of GnRH (gonadotropin releasing hormone) you would see that levels went up and down in a saw-tooth manner over short periods of time. Overall, the pattern of secretion for hormones which are secreted episodically depends on other factors such as the half-life of the hormone and the frequency and amplitude of secretory episodes.

Diurnal variation

The secretion of many hormones has a predictable daily pattern which is known as diurnal variation (see Fig. 1.10). Growth hormone concentrations, for example, are usually so low that they are undetectable during the day, but increase during the early part of sleep. In contrast, corticotropin concentrations are at their lowest at midnight and reach a peak at around 0800h each day. It is clearly important to be aware of diurnal variation when circulating hormone levels are being measured.

The main regulator of the 24-h periodicity of hormone secretion is the 'body clock', principally the suprachiasmatic nucleus (SCN) in the hypothalamus. However, other factors can influence the diurnal pattern of secretion. For example, cortisol, which increases in response to food intake, also increases in anticipation shortly before the times when we normally eat. Melatonin is one of the most obviously day–night related hormones. Its secretion is suppressed by light so it is produced during the hours of darkness (see Ch. 13). There is also evidence from cell culture experiments which suggests that some endocrine cells may even have their own inbuilt 24-h clock to help control their diurnal secretion.

Set point regulation

It is quite unusual for a hormone to be maintained at a set level. However, thyroxine concentrations in blood vary very little from day to day and are constant within a 24-h period. Changes in thyroxine concentrations occur only over weeks or months. One reason for this is the very long half-life of thyroxine in blood.

Different hormones clearly have markedly different patterns of secretion. However, most have some diurnal pattern but with episodic secretion on top of this underlying rhythm. Thus, there is a daily rhythm plus an element of response to physiological demand in the final pattern of secretion of most hormones.

Endocrine axis

Many hormones function as part of a cascade, so that the target tissue of one hormone is another endocrine gland. For example, thyrotropin releasing hormone (TRH) from the hypothalamus stimulates the release of pituitary TSH, which in turn stimulates release of thyroxine from the thyroid. The cascade allows amplifications of signal, flexibility of response to a variety of physiological stimuli and fine regulation of levels of the end hormonal product. This functional grouping is called an endocrine axis (Fig. 1.11) and, in the example we have used is called the hypothalamo–pituitary–thyroid axis. There are examples of endocrine axes in most of the following chapters.

Negative feedback

One of the most important principles of endocrine regulation is the concept of negative feedback. We have seen that one of the functions of hormones is to regulate homeostatic mechanisms in the body. However, there is also a homeostatic process that regulates levels of hormones. Basically, the body has systems which are designed to 'damp-down' excess of any kind. The simplest form of

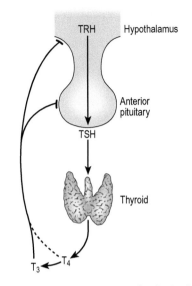

Figure 1.11 An endocrine axis and negative feedback. The axis shown is the hypothalamo–pituitary–thyroid axis. Thyrotropin releasing hormone (TRH), from the hypothalamus, stimulates the release of thyroid stimulating hormone (TSH) from the anterior pituitary. The TSH stimulates the thyroid gland to release T_4 and T_3, which exert a negative feedback inhibitory effect on the hypothalamus and pituitary glands.

negative feedback is where the final product of an endocrine cascade acts to inhibit release of hormones higher up the cascade (see Fig. 1.11). In the example shown, a stimulus such as exercise causes an increase in thyrotropin releasing hormone (TRH) from the hypothalamus, which in turn acts to increase the secretion of thyroid stimulating hormone (TSH) from the anterior pituitary. The increased TSH stimulates the thyroid gland to produce thyroxine but one of the effects of thyroxine is to act on both the hypothalamus and anterior pituitary to decrease the production of TRH and TSH, respectively. This pattern, of the final product of a cascade system exerting negative feedback higher up the endocrine axis, is one which you will see repeated throughout this book.

Negative feedback does not mean that hormone production is switched on and off like a light switch. There is a basal or residual rate of hormone secretion which can be increased by a variety of stimuli and decreased by negative feedback. This means that all endocrine systems are dynamic, in other words they are responsive to change and with a tendency to return to the basal or residual state of activity.

Most negative feedback operates through a genomic mechanism resulting in a decrease in the production of hormones higher up the endocrine axis. This process takes place over a relatively long time period, hours to days, and so it is known as 'delayed feedback'. An example of this would be the action of thyroxine on the production of TRH and TSH. This type of feedback is determined by both the amplitude of the original increase in hormone secretion and its duration.

Some systems also have a more rapid negative feedback response called 'fast feedback', which is clearly not mediated by a genomic mechanism as it can take place within ten minutes. For example, in the hypothalamo–pituitary–adrenal axis, the hormonal end-product is cortisol. If cortisol levels rise rapidly, this triggers a fast feedback mechanism which reduces activity of the axis at higher levels. The speed of this response suggests that cortisol exerts its fast feedback effect through a different mechanism than the conventional genomic mechanism of steroid action. So in general, fast feedback kicks in when hormone levels rise rapidly and is triggered by the gradient of the increase. Delayed feedback, in contrast, is determined by the amplitude and duration of the end-product response and takes place over longer time periods.

So far, we have only considered those feedback loops from the end-products of an endocrine cascade. The hormones that exert this form of negative feedback effect are usually small molecules that can readily cross the blood–brain barrier, as the hypothalamus is an important site of negative feedback in many hormone systems. Some systems also have short feedback loops which allow intermediate products of an endocrine axis to exert negative feedback at higher levels. For example pituitary corticotropin (ACTH), which stimulates cortisol secretion, also inhibits hypothalamic corticotropin releasing hormone (CRH). This suggests that there are specific mechanisms to allow transport of certain peptide hormones across the blood–brain barrier.

So, in summary, the CRH–ACTH–cortisol cascade is regulated by both classical negative feedback from cortisol (the end-product) and by short-loop feedback from ACTH (the intermediate product).

The principle of negative feedback is the basis of several dynamic tests of endocrine function. The general principle is that failure of high levels of a hormone to be suppressed by its negative feedback regulator suggests that there is a pathological abnormality in the system. Specific examples are given throughout this book.

Hormone antagonism and synergy

When a hormone has an effect, it is called an agonist. A hormone which has the opposite effect is said to be an antagonist of the first hormone (see Ch. 2 for details of agonists and antagonists).

In cases where it is really important to maintain the levels of a substance within narrow limits, the body takes a 'belt and braces' approach and uses more than one hormone to achieve the control. Very often, the hormones will act in opposition: one or more will tend to increase the level of the substance, while one or more will act to decrease it. This might seem wasteful, but it has two very important consequences. One is that it allows considerable fine control and responsiveness to a changing environment. The second is that it can afford protection against a potentially devastating change in the level of the substance. For example, there are many hormones involved in glucose homeostasis. However, only one of these, insulin, acts to decrease blood glucose levels, while all the rest act as insulin antagonists and increase blood glucose levels. The interactions between them allow fine control and the number of hormones which increase glucose helps to protect against potentially fatal hypoglycaemia.

Sometimes, hormones which exert the same effect have much greater action when the two act together than either of them can have individually. This is called synergy and is rare in endocrine systems. The best example is the synergy between CRH and AVP in stimulating ACTH secretion (see Ch. 4).

Endocrine disorders

As a general rule, endocrine disorders are the result of either excessive secretion of a hormone or of insufficient secretion. The terminology used to describe these disorders can be confusing. Too much hormone is indicated by the prefix *hyper-*, while too little hormone is indicated by the prefix *hypo-* (from the Greek meaning 'over' and 'below', respectively). So hypercortisolism is the state of excess cortisol production. The suffix can also change to indicate where the excess occurs, so hypercortisolaemia is too much cortisol in the blood. Glycosuria means that there is glucose in the urine. In this case we do not need to use hypo- or hyper-, because glucose is not normally found in urine, so the fact of its presence is all that needs reporting.

The effects of either hormone excess or relative absence of hormone are exaggerations of the normal physiological effects of the hormone and serve as a very useful illustration of endocrine physiology. Historically, endocrine disease states were used to gain an understanding of the actions of different hormones. The cases used in this book have been chosen to illustrate important points about either the biochemistry of hormone synthesis or the physiology of endocrine regulation. The common endocrine disorders are listed in Table 1.5 according to the chapter in which you will find them described.

The endocrine axes described above mean that a deficiency in the final hormone of the cascade may be due to a defect at one of several points in the axis. Looking at the example of an endocrine axis shown in Figure 1.11, a defect in the thyroid gland itself would result in primary thyroid failure, a problem with pituitary secretion of TSH would be called secondary thyroid failure, and a deficiency of TRH from the hypothalamus would be called tertiary thyroid failure. This categorization of primary, secondary and tertiary defect is generally used in describing disorders of an endocrine axis. Another generalizable feature is that very often the symptoms of the disorder may be similar for each of the primary, secondary and tertiary causes because they all result in abnormal secretion of the final hormone in the axis.

We started the Preface to this book with Professor John Landon's quote about clinical endocrinology being about either too much or too little of a hormone. As you may have guessed however, endocrinology is a bit more

Table 1.5 Endocrine disorders described in this book: their major features and the chapter where you can read about them

Name	Cause	Ch.	Features
Common, likely to be seen in a GP surgery			
Cushing's syndrome	Excess glucocorticoid (any cause)	6	Central obesity, hypertension, IGT, 'moon-face', bruising, osteoporosis
Goitre	Growth of thyroid gland	7	Thyroid hormone secretion may be high, low or normal
Hyperthyroidism	Increased T3/T4 any cause	7	Weight loss, heat intolerance, increased heart rate, tremor, anxiety
Hypothyroidism	Decreased T3/T4 any cause	7	Weight gain, cold intolerance, muscle weakness, decreased heart rate, depression
Hypogonadism	Any cause: men decreased testosterone	8	Infertility, impotence, decreased secondary sex characteristics
	Women decreased oestrogen	9	Absent periods. Infertility, osteoporosis
Polycystic ovarian syndrome (PCOS)	Increased androgens in women	9	Abnormal periods, decreased fertility, hirsutism, obesity, IGT
Menopause	↓ Oestrogen at end of reproductive life	10	Periods stop, infertile, flushes, sweats, osteoporosis
Diabetes mellitus	Type 1 lack of insulin secretion	11	Weight loss, thirst, ↑ urine production, ketoacidosis, long term organ damage
	Type 2 insulin receptor insensitivity	11	Obesity, thirst, ↑ urine production, cardiovascular disease
Metabolic syndrome	Insulin resistance	11	Combination of obesity, IGT, hypertension, ↑ cholesterol
Commonly seen in a specialist endocrine clinic			
Ectopic hormone secretion	Hormone secretion by tumour cells	1	Depends on hormone secreted
Diabetes insipidus	Cranial, failure of AVP secretion	3	Failure to concentrate urine, dehydration
	Nephrogenic, many causes	3	
SIADH	↑ AVP	3	Inappropriate water retention, low plasma sodium
Acromegaly	↑ Growth hormone in adult	4	Growth of soft tissues and viscera, IGT
Hyperprolactinaemia	↑ Prolactin	4	Women, stop periods, lactation
			Men, breast development, milk production
Panhypopituitarism	↓ In anterior pituitary hormones	4	Features of ↓ GH, LH/FSH, ACTH and TSH.
Phaeochromocytoma	↑ Adrenaline and noradrenaline	5	Raised blood pressure, ↑ heart rate, anxiety
Congenital adrenal hyperplasia	Abnormal adrenal steroid secretion	6	Children: failure to thrive, virilization of girls
Addison's disease	Primary adrenal insufficiency ↓ cortisol	6	Weakness, hypotension, dehydration, ↓ sodium ↑ potassium
Grave's disease	Autoimmune cause of ↑ T3/T4	7	As hypothyroid with exophthalmos and myxoedema
Hashimoto's thyroiditis	Autoimmune cause of ↓ T3/T4	7	As hypothyroid
Klinefelter's syndrome	Chromosomal abnormality XXY	8, 10	Male hypogonadism
Turner's syndrome	Chromosomal abnormality X0	10	Female absent puberty, periods do not start, infertility, cardiovascular abnormalities
Premature ovarian failure	↓ Oestrogen, menopause before 40	10	As menopause
Hyperparathyroidism	Primary ↑ PTH	12	Hypercalcaemia, (stones, moans, groans), dehydration
	Ectopic ↑ PTHrp	12	
Osteomalacia	Vitamin D deficiency in adults	12	↓ Bone density, pathological fractures
Rarely seen, even in a specialist endocrine clinic			
Giantism	↑ Growth hormone in children	4	Increased growth, especially height in childhood
Laron syndrome	Abnormal growth hormone receptor	4	Decreased growth in childhood

(Continued)

Table 1.5 Continued

Name	Cause	Ch.	Features
Sheehan syndrome	Disrupted blood flow to pituitary	4	As panhypopituitarism
Cushing's disease	↑ ACTH from pituitary	6	As Cushing's syndrome
Conn's syndrome	Excess aldosterone	6	Hypertension, low serum potassium
Cretinism	↓ T3/T4 in utero or congenital hypothyroidism	7	Severe mental retardation
Kallmann's syndrome	Cause of male tertiary hypogonadism	8	As hypogonadism with anosmia
Anabolic androgenic steroid abuse	↓ Testosterone	8	Infertility, male testicular atrophy, aggression, women virilization
Rickets	Vitamin D deficiency in children	12	↓ Bone mineralization, bone deformities
Hypoparathyroidism	↓ PTH	12	Hypocalcaemia, pins and needles, tetany, convulsions
Zollinger–Ellison syndrome	↑ Gastrin	13	Severe peptic ulceration
Multiple endocrine neoplasia	Various	13	Tumours of different endocrine glands

IGT, impaired glucose tolerance.

complicated than that. While most endocrine disorders are the result of either excessive secretion of a hormone or of insufficient secretion, there are also a number of clinical conditions which result from receptor insensitivity to a hormone. A good example of this is non-insulin dependent diabetes (see Ch. 11), which can be considered to be a condition of insulin resistance. In other words, although there is circulating insulin and there are insulin receptors on the target cells, it does not have the same effectiveness.

Endocrine investigations: general principles

The investigation of endocrine disorders usually starts with a simple single-point measurement of plasma hormone concentrations. In some cases, this measurement may be sufficient to determine whether there is a disorder, but when the hormone under investigation is secreted episodically (such as growth hormone or cortisol), a single-point measurement is often of very limited value. In this case, a *dynamic test* of the endocrine system is used. The principle of dynamic testing is really quite simple: when an excess of hormone is suspected, the aim of the dynamic test is to suppress hormone levels. If, on the other hand, insufficient secretion is suspected, then the aim of the test is to stimulate secretion. As far as possible the tests aim to check the whole system.

There are two general reasons for performing endocrine investigations (Box 1.1). The first is to confirm a diagnosis and the second is to monitor the progress of a disease. There are a large number of possible tests aimed at confirming a diagnosis, and so a degree of selection and judgement has to be introduced. The selection of

Box 1.1 Endocrine tests

- Tests may be for purposes of diagnosis or monitoring
- Diagnostic tests may be selected after clinical pattern recognition or by understanding basic principles of physiology and anatomy
- Blood tests may be basal or dynamic
- Basal tests are usually at 0900h in a fasted state
- In dynamic testing: select a stimulation test if a hormone level is suspected of being too low, but a suppression test if the level is suspected of being too high.

tests to perform must be guided by the clinical situation, and here the clinician may use two types of approach. One approach is to make a clinical diagnosis based on pattern recognition. For example, a classical combination of symptoms in endocrine disease is weight loss despite a good appetite (seen in thyrotoxicosis), which will lead an experienced clinician into testing the thyroid gland. A second approach is to use the basic principles of physiology and anatomy in guiding diagnostic testing. This is needed if the clinical pattern is unclear or a surprising result is found. For example, a patient may be found to have atrial fibrillation (an irregular heart rhythm) when undergoing a routine examination before an operation. As high thyroid hormone levels stimulate the heart, and in particular the atrial chambers, this should lead to thyroid function testing, even in the absence of other classical symptoms.

The most commonly used tests in endocrinology measure hormones and minerals in blood samples (Box 1.2). The levels of most hormones vary through the day and

Box 1.2 Measurement of hormones

As hormones circulate in such small concentrations, measuring hormone levels in blood presents a particular challenge. Original assay methods used the biological response to a hormone to estimate the amount present and were termed 'bioassays'. An example is the early pregnancy test which relied on the observation that human chorionic gonadotropin (hCG), the level of which is raised in early pregnancy, causes the female *Xenopus* toad to ovulate. These assays had the advantage that they measured only biologically active hormone. However, they had several disadvantages: they were often relatively insensitive and they usually used animals or animal tissues. This not only raised ethical issues, but also made the assays inherently unreliable because of the variability of the response. Modern methods of hormone assay usually use a competitive binding assay, such as a radioimmunoassay, which is very sensitive (Fig. 1.12). These have been developed to a level of sophistication that makes them simple to perform, rapid and very reliable. It is now possible to purchase kits that measure all the known hormones at the concentrations found in human plasma.

A specific antibody is needed

The antibody is chemically bound to a solid surface

The sample containing the hormone (H) is added to the surface

Two methods are used:

1 Single-site competitive assay
(for small-sized hormones)

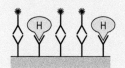

The antibody binds the hormones

A competitor for the antibody is added and binds free sites. The competitor is labelled and emits a signal that can be measured

The amount of hormone is deduced from the total antibody sites minus free sites

2 Two-site non-competitive assay
(for large-sized hormones)

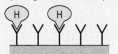

The antibody binds the hormones

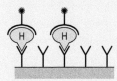

A different antibody binds the hormone at a second site. The second antibody is labelled and measured

Figure 1.12 Measurement of hormones in blood by immunoassay.

the normal ranges are very dependent on the time a sample is taken; thus, normal ranges are usually based on samples taken at 0900 hours and in a fasted state. It is vital to the correct interpretation of a blood test result that the time of the sample is recorded. These samples are also known as basal samples as they represent the base, or unstimulated, state. Samples are also tested at specific times after stimulation or suppression and these are called dynamic tests. An example is the stimulation of the steroid hormone cortisol from the adrenal gland 30 and 60 min after an injection of synthetic adrenocorticotropin.

The maximum information is obtained when a hormone and its regulator are measured together. For example, if thyroxine and TSH are measured together then it is immediately clear whether the disease process is in the thyroid or the pituitary.

Interesting fact

In clinical endocrinology, as in other branches of medicine, it is fairly unusual for a patient to present with every single classical symptom and sign of a particular condition (with no red herrings). Such a case is called 'textbook' or a 'textbook example' because they are rarely encountered outside the pages of books.

Biological samples

All blood, urine and biopsy samples need to be collected in the correct containers. Some hormones have a very short life and a falsely low value may occur if the procedure is not done properly. For example, adrenocorticotropin has a half-life in the blood of about 10 min, so the blood must be taken in a chilled syringe and bottle, and then the plasma has to be separated immediately from blood by centrifugation.

Urine testing is very important in endocrinology. A simple stick can be dipped into urine and chemical pads will detect the presence of glucose (suggesting diabetes), blood, protein, white cells, ketones, acidity and even hormones (e.g. hCG, indicating pregnancy). This yields a tremendous amount of clinical information and a dip-stick test should be performed in all new patients. Hormones and minerals are usually best measured in accurately timed 24-h urine samples. All urine produced over this time is placed in a bottle and the total excretion of a hormone can be measured.

Imaging

Radiological imaging is vital to the assessment of endocrine glands. The type of test selected depends on the gland (Table 1.6). For example, the pituitary is surrounded by a bony cup and is not well seen by radiography. The best image is obtained with magnetic resonance imaging.

Table 1.6 Imaging and endocrine glands

Gland	Imaging modality
Pituitary and hypothalamus	Magnetic resonance imaging (MRI)
Adrenal	CT initially
Pancreas	CT initially
Thyroid	Ultrasonography
Testes	Ultrasonography
Ovaries	Ultrasonography (transvaginal)

Ectopic hormone secretion

It is not only the well-defined endocrine tissues that can secrete hormones. All cells retain the genetic capacity for hormone secretion and it is increasingly recognized that malignant cells may express the genes encoding hormonally active peptides. As the usual mechanism for hormone processing is not usually present in these malignancies, the peptide secreted may be a fragment or a precursor of the normal mature hormone. The inappropriate secretion of hormones by tissues that do not usually produce that hormone is called 'ectopic' hormone secretion. Often ectopic hormone secretion is seen as a feature of endocrine tumours; for example, pancreatic islet cell carcinomas have occasionally been found to secrete adrenocorticotropic hormone (ACTH), which usually comes from the pituitary gland. Non-endocrine tissues may also secrete hormones; for example, inappropriate ACTH secretion is a recognized feature of some small cell carcinomas of the lung.

The most common example of ectopic hormone secretion is a peptide hormone called parathyroid hormone-related peptide (PTHrp), which is secreted by around 10% of malignant tumours and causes hypercalcaemia, termed 'hypercalcaemia of malignancy'.

Ectopic hormone secretion is diagnosed through a combined approach of imaging, together with arterio-venous sampling to measure a hormone concentration gradient across a tissue and so establish the source of the hormone.

Interesting fact

Endocrine disorders can have such profound effects on the body that many disorders are 'foot of the bed' diagnoses. You will read about the characteristic changes of acromegaly, Cushing's syndrome, Graves' disease and hypothyroidism later. All of these disorders of hormone secretion result in changes to the appearance that makes it possible to recognize them from a distance. Keep your eyes open on the bus!

RECEPTORS AND HORMONE ACTION

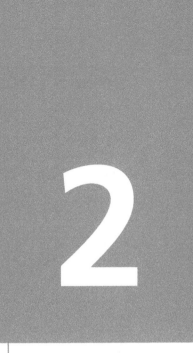

Chapter objectives

After studying this chapter you should be able to:

1. Understand that hormones exert their effects by binding to specific receptors in target tissues.

2. Explain what is meant by receptor specificity and affinity and by ligand potency and efficacy.

3. Explain the significance of receptor agonists and antagonists.

4. Categorize common hormones by the types of receptor they bind to.

5. Understand how hormone binding to a receptor brings about changes in cellular activity.

6. Understand the role of second messengers and protein kinases in hormone action.

Introduction

All hormones act by binding to receptors in their target cells and by doing so bring about an intracellular response. It is the presence of receptors, which are highly specific binding proteins, that defines the target cells for a hormone: target cells of a hormone are those cells that have receptors for the hormone. The location of these receptors in each cell depends to some extent on the chemical nature of the hormone. Peptide hormones act on receptors located in the cell membrane, while steroid hormones act on intracellular receptors. There are many forms of receptor and several different ways in which the action of a hormone binding to a receptor can cause a change in intracellular activity. In this chapter we shall explore the many different forms of hormone action.

General characteristics of receptors

Receptor agonists and antagonists

A receptor is a specialized protein, located in the cell membrane, cytoplasm or nucleus of a target cell, which acts to pass on a chemical message. Receptors have binding sites to receive the message and the effect of this interaction is to bring about changes in the receptor which result in the message being passed on to initiate a cellular response. Although the receptor has a 'specific binding site' for the physiological chemical message, receptors will usually bind any compound which is structurally similar to the message. Any compound which binds to a receptor is called a 'ligand' for that receptor. So a hormone is a naturally occurring ligand for its target cell receptor.

However, not all ligands will bring about the normal conformational changes in the receptor. Ligands which bind to the receptor but do not initiate the cellular response are called 'antagonists' because they block the normal function of the receptor. Ligands which do initiate the cellular response are called 'agonists', so hormones are agonists at their receptors. Both receptor agonists and antagonists are often used pharmacologically to mimic or to block the effects of hormones.

Let's think of some examples. Cortisol (a naturally occurring glucocorticoid hormone), methylprednisolone (a synthetic glucocorticoid) and mifepristone (an anti-glucocorticoid drug) all bind to the glucocorticoid receptor. Both cortisol and methylprednisolone are agonists and induce a cellular response by activating the glucocorticoid receptor. Mifepristone is an antagonist which binds to the glucocorticoid receptor but does not pass on the normal message and so can be used to block the effects of circulating glucocorticoids.

Dose–response effects

A feature of a receptor-mediated effect is that is has dose–response characteristics (Fig. 2.1): the response increases

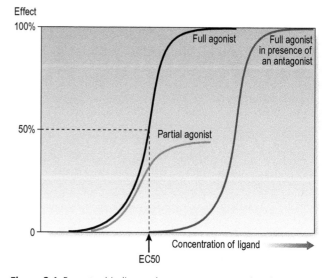

Figure 2.1 Receptor binding: a dose–response curve showing a typical sigmoid shape of increasing effect with increasing ligand concentration. A partial agonist never produces the same magnitude of effect, even at maximal concentrations. The presence of an antagonist has the effect of moving the dose–response curve to the right so that a higher concentration of agonist is required to produce the same effect, but the same maximal effect is still achievable.

with increasing amounts of the hormone, until a plateau is reached. At the plateau the receptor system is saturated. The dose–response curves are used to investigate the effects of agonists and antagonists at the receptor. In the presence of some antagonists, a higher concentration of the hormone is required to elicit the effect.

A drug or hormone that is a partial agonist at a receptor elicits a lesser maximal response than a full agonist at that receptor (Fig. 2.1).

Receptor binding properties

Receptors have two important binding characteristics, affinity and specificity. Binding affinity relates to how tightly the hormone binds the receptor while specificity refers to whether the receptor binds just one hormone or whether it might bind other closely related molecules. This is particularly relevant when we are looking at steroid receptors where the steroid hormones are structurally very similar.

A receptor needs to have a high affinity for the hormone in order to bind to it. However, hormone binding to a receptor is a reversible process and in an equilibrium the hormone and receptor constantly associate and dissociate. Because of the law of mass action:

[receptor-ligand complex] = [unbound ligand] [unbound receptor].

The dissociation constant, K_D, for the receptor is defined as:

$$\frac{[\text{unbound receptor}]\,[\text{unbound ligand}]}{[\text{receptor-ligand complex}]}$$

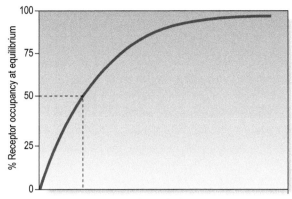

Figure 2.2 Dissociation constant. The dissociation constant is the concentration of ligand at which half the receptor sites are occupied when the reaction is at equilibrium. This is derived experimentally by incubating a sample containing receptors with increasing quantities of radiolabelled ligand. At equilibrium the bound ligand is separated from the free ligand and a saturation curve of increasing receptor occupancy such as this is obtained.

This means that K_D is the concentration of ligand when half the receptors are occupied, as [unbound receptor] and [receptor-ligand complex] will then be the same and cancel each other out. So K_D is measured by the concentration of hormone required to produce 50% receptor occupancy; and affinity is defined as $1/K_D$ (Fig. 2.2) and high affinity means a low K_D.

Interesting fact

The usual analogy for receptors and ligands is a lock and a big bunch of keys. Several keys (ligands) might fit into the lock (receptor) but only one or two keys (agonists) are likely to open it. Keys which fit but do not open the lock have the effect of blocking the receptor (antagonists).

Of course, this rather simplistic analogy breaks down for partial agonists. These compounds are particularly fascinating because they bind to the receptor and activate it, but the cellular response is less than that produced by a 'full agonist'. In the presence of a full agonist, a partial agonist will compete for binding sites and reduce the normal cellular response, in other words it can also have antagonist effects. You will come across several examples of partial agonists in this book.

To add another level of complexity, conventional pharmacology assumes that each receptor is only linked to one system which passes on the message. However, membrane receptors, which can move around in a fluid membrane, may associate with more than one second messenger or other signalling system. So different ligands binding to the same receptor can activate different signalling pathways within the cell. This situation, where different cellular responses triggered by a receptor are ligand-dependent is known as 'functional selectivity'. Going back to our lock and key analogy, it is as if one lock could open any of several different doors, depending on which key you use!

Hormones circulate in very low concentrations indeed. The lower the concentration of a hormone, the higher the receptor affinity needs to be in order to elicit a response. Most receptor's K_D for its hormone is therefore very low, typically in the picomolar range.

Ligand properties

Two properties of ligands that are particularly important in pharmacology are efficacy and potency. Efficacy is a measure of the amount of bound ligand required to produce a given response. A ligand with a high efficacy will produce a large response even when it has occupied only a small number of binding sites. In contrast, a ligand with low efficacy will need to occupy a high proportion of binding sites to elicit the same response, and a partial agonist, even with all the binding sites occupied, will elicit a sub-maximal response.

Potency is a measure of the concentration of ligand required to produce a given response. A ligand with high potency will produce a large response even at low concentrations. The measure of potency is called the EC50, the concentration of a ligand required to produce a half-maximal response (Fig. 2.1). The more potent the ligand, the lower the EC50.

As you will have noted, efficacy and potency are related to each other via affinity.

Types of hormone receptors

There are three major classes of hormone receptor: G-protein coupled receptors; kinase-linked receptors (both located in the plasma membrane of the cell); and intracellular receptors. Table 2.1 shows the major classes of receptors and the hormones which interact with each type. We shall consider each of these receptor types in turn, looking first at the two types of cell-membrane receptor.

Cell-membrane receptors

Peptides, glycoproteins and catecholamines are either too large or too hydrophilic to enter the cell and so these hormones bind to receptors located in the plasma membrane, with their ligand binding domain (hormone binding site) on the extracellular surface. There are two broad classes of cell surface receptor: those which are G-protein coupled and act through the generation of a second messenger and those that directly activate a protein kinase.

G-protein coupled receptors (GPCRs) and second messengers

This group of receptors is probably the most widespread through the endocrine system. Receptors are linked via G-protein activation to second messenger production or ion channel opening (Fig. 2.3).

Table 2.1 Major receptor subtypes and the hormones that interact with them

Cell surface receptors	
G-protein coupled receptors	Many peptide hormones including ACTH, TSH, LH, FSH, vasopressin, oxytocin, glucagon, PTH
	Catecholamines
Receptors with inbuilt kinase activity	Insulin and growth factors
Receptors which directly activate kinases	Growth hormone, prolactin, cytokines
Intracellular receptors	
Type 1: Steroid hormone receptors	Cortisol, aldosterone, testosterone, oestradiol, progesterone
Type 2: Nuclear receptors	Thyroxine, calcitriol

Table 2.2 Types of G-proteins and their major actions

Type	**Action**
Gs (alpha s)	Activates adenylyl cyclase
	Opens calcium channels in some tissues
Gq (alpha q)	Activates phospholipase C
Gi (alpha i)	Inhibits adenylyl cyclase

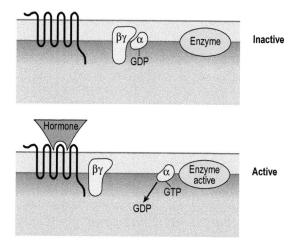

Figure 2.4 G-protein interactions with a seven transmembrane domain receptor. In the absence of hormone binding the G-protein subunits are associated and the α subunit binds GDP. When the hormone binds to the receptor a conformational change causes the α subunit to bind GTP instead of GDP and to move away from the βγ units. The α subunit is then able to exert an effect on an enzyme or ion channel. Inbuilt hydrolase activity converts the GTP to GDP which inactivates the α subunit causing it to return to the basal state.

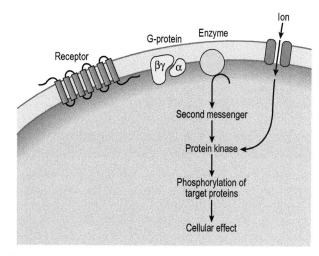

Figure 2.3 G-protein coupled receptor signalling by generation of a second messenger or opening of an ion channel.

The receptor protein spans the cell membrane with seven helices, an external N-terminal and an intracellular C-terminal. These receptors are also called seven transmembrane domain receptors. The receptor, when occupied, can interact with a protein on the intracellular face of the cell membrane, called a G-protein (Fig. 2.4). A G-protein consists of three distinct subunits, termed alpha, beta and gamma. The beta and gamma subunits are constant but many different forms of the alpha subunit exist and these different forms interact with different targets, either enzymes or ion channels. A summary of the different forms of alpha subunit and their effects is shown in Table 2.2.

In the resting state, the three G-protein subunits are physically close to each other and the alpha subunit binds guanosine diphosphate (GDP). It is the guanosine binding capability that gives G-proteins their name. When the hormone binds to the seven transmembrane domain

receptors it causes the receptor to change shape, known as inducing a conformational change in the protein (Fig. 2.4). That shape change causes the G-protein to drop the GDP and bind a GTP molecule instead. The alpha subunit, with its bound GTP, separates from the beta and gamma subunits and moves through the membrane to interact with its target protein. When it comes adjacent to the target, such as the enzyme adenylyl cyclase, it causes a conformational change in the enzyme, which activates it. In this way the G-protein is the signal transduction mechanism which passes the signal from the receptor to stimulate production of a second messenger.

Once it has been activated, how is the enzyme switched off? The signal from the G-protein is stopped when the alpha subunit is no longer bound to GTP. The alpha subunit possesses GTP-ase activity which breaks down the GTP into GDP and it is this which returns the alpha subunit to its inactive form, so that it diffuses back through the membrane to associate with the beta and gamma subunits. In the absence of the activated alpha subunit the enzyme returns to its inactive form and stops producing second messengers.

Interesting fact

Cholera is an ancient disease, known for hundreds of years, which still causes many deaths in periodic outbreaks today. It is a severe form of diarrhoea which rapidly causes dehydration and death, sometimes in as little as 4 hours after symptoms start. It is caused by a bacterium, *Vibrio cholerae*, which is spread by faecal contamination of drinking water, and the discovery of the epidemiology of cholera is one of the great stories of Victorian medicine. The mechanism by which *Vibrio cholerae* brings about its effects has only been fully described in the past 30 years and it involves G-proteins.

The A-subunit of the cholera toxin enters the enterocyte (gut cell) and causes a covalent modification (ADP-ribosylation) of the alpha subunit of a G-protein, Gs. This causes the alpha subunit to lose its GTP-ase activity so it cannot turn itself off. It also causes the alpha subunit to dissociate from the beta-gamma units much more readily and it prevents the alpha subunit from dissociating from adenylyl cyclase. The net effect of all this is that the alpha subunit causes a prolonged stimulation of adenylyl cyclase, with a huge rise in intracellular cAMP. Acting via protein kinase A, this results in the phosphorylation of chloride ion channels on the luminal membrane of the enterocytes. Chloride ions leak into the gut lumen, followed by sodium, moving down the electrochemical gradient. The influx of ions into the lumen of the gut takes water with it, resulting in the formation of a large volume of isotonic diarrhoea. Dehydration is rapid. And all because a G-protein got locked in the activated state.

Second messenger systems

A range of compounds are employed by cells to act as 'second messengers'. These are chemical signals that relay the hormonal signal (the first messenger) within the cell. The common feature of second messengers is that they all have a very short half-life within the cell and are deactivated very rapidly by either chemical degradation or by re-uptake.

Cyclic AMP

The commonest second messenger is cyclic adenosine monophosphate (cAMP, Fig. 2.5). This is produced by the dephosphorylation of ATP by the enzyme adenylyl cyclase which is located in the cell membrane. Some GPCRs activate adenylyl cyclase while others, acting through alpha i, inhibit cAMP production (Table 2.2). Within the cell, cAMP acts by binding to protein kinase A (see Fig. 2.8). Intracellular cAMP is rapidly broken down by phosphodiesterase.

Phosphatidylinositol bisphosphate

Another second messenger system is activated when the GPCR is coupled to activation of phospholipase C (Fig. 2.6). This enzyme cleaves a membrane phospholipid, phosphatidylinositol bisphosphate (PIP_2) to give two second messengers, inositol trisphosphate (IP_3) and

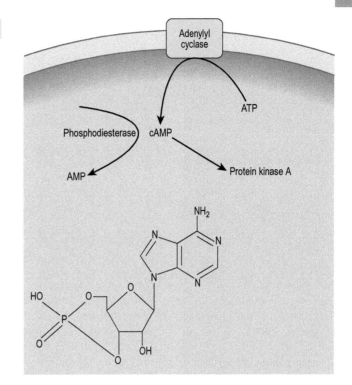

Figure 2.5 Cell signalling through cAMP: formation, actions and breakdown of cAMP.

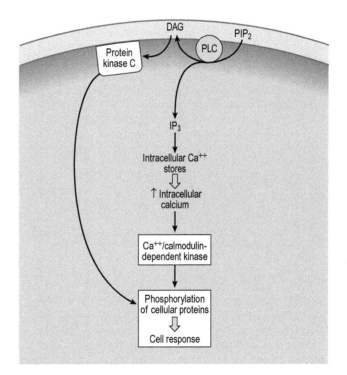

Figure 2.6 Signalling through IP_3 and DAG.

diacylglycerol (DAG) (Fig. 2.7). The DAG remains in the cell membrane where it attracts and activates protein kinase C. The IP_3 is an important component of calcium signalling.

RECEPTORS AND HORMONE ACTION

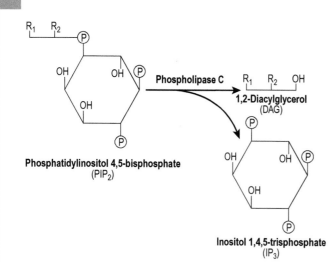

Figure 2.7 Actions of phospholipase C (PLC). PLC cleaves phosphatidylinositol bisphosphate into diacylglycerol (DAG) and inositol 1,4,5, trisphosphate (IP$_3$). R$_1$ is usually stearate and R$_2$ is usually arachidonate. IP$_3$ is inactivated by dephosphorylation.

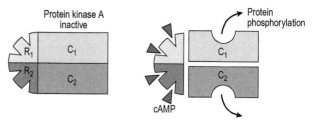

Figure 2.8 Signalling through cAMP: interaction with protein kinase A (PKA). The PKA consists of four subunits, two regulatory (R$_1$ and R$_2$) and two catalytic (C$_1$ and C$_2$). In the absence of cAMP these are closely associated. When cAMP binds to the sites on the regulatory subunits, the four units dissociate, which activates the catalytic subunits.

Calcium signalling

There are two elements to calcium signalling: first is the G-protein-dependent opening of ligand gated ion channels in the cell membrane, allowing an influx of calcium into the cell. The second is release of intracellular calcium stores, mediated by release of IP$_3$ by the actions of phospholipase C (above). The IP$_3$ remains within the cytoplasm and acts to open calcium channels in the endoplasmic reticulum causing the release of calcium into the cytoplasm (Fig. 2.6). Together these two mechanisms cause increases in the cytoplasmic calcium concentration. Calcium acts as a second messenger, activating calcium/calmodulin dependent protein kinase.

Interesting fact

The second messenger cyclic AMP is not just found in mammalian cells. It is produced and secreted by slime moulds, where it acts as a signalling molecule, enabling communication between individual cells.

Protein kinases and phosphatases

You will have noted, reading the section above on second messengers, that second messengers commonly act through protein kinases to influence intracellular events. Protein kinases are regulatory proteins which bind the second messenger and then phosphorylate target proteins in the cell, usually enzymes, either activating or inactivating them by phosphorylation.

Protein kinase A, also known as cAMP-dependent protein kinase is perhaps the best characterized of all these. It consists of two regulatory subunits and two catalytic subunits (Fig. 2.8). When cAMP binds to the regulatory subunits they undergo a conformational change and

separate from the catalytic subunits. This physical separation causes activation of the two catalytic subunits which then phosphorylate serine and threonine residues on specific cellular proteins. When the bound cAMP dissociates from the binding sites on the regulatory subunits the kinase reassembles itself and the catalytic activity stops.

Phosphorylation of these cellular proteins, usually enzymes, causes either activation or deactivation of the enzyme. This is reversed by the action of cellular phosphatases, which dephosphorylate the protein, returning the cellular activity to its basal state. An example of a cellular protein which is activated in response to phosphorylation by protein kinase A is cholesterol ester hydrolase (a hormone-sensitive lipase), which acts to liberate cholesterol in steroidogenic cells in preparation for steroid biosynthesis.

Receptor desensitization and downregulation: GPKs and beta arrestin

When a hormone binds to a G-protein coupled receptor the receptor is usually quickly de-sensitized and eventually internalized within the cell for subsequent breakdown or recycling. The first step of this process involves two families of intracellular proteins which, like the G-proteins, are able to interact with all members of this receptor family. These are the beta arrestins and the G-protein coupled receptor kinases (GPK) (Fig. 2.9). Hormone binding to a receptor causes interaction of the receptor with G-proteins as we have seen above. It also attracts an enzyme of the GPK family which phosphorylates the receptor. The phosphorylated receptor has a lower binding affinity for the hormone but also attracts beta arrestin binding, which physically blocks interaction of the receptor with G-proteins and so prevents further signalling through second messengers.

The desensitized receptors then move through the plasma membrane to accumulate in clathrin-coated pits (specialized areas of the cell membrane involved in endocytosis) which become internalized within the cell. The beta arrestin has a further role in recruiting proteins

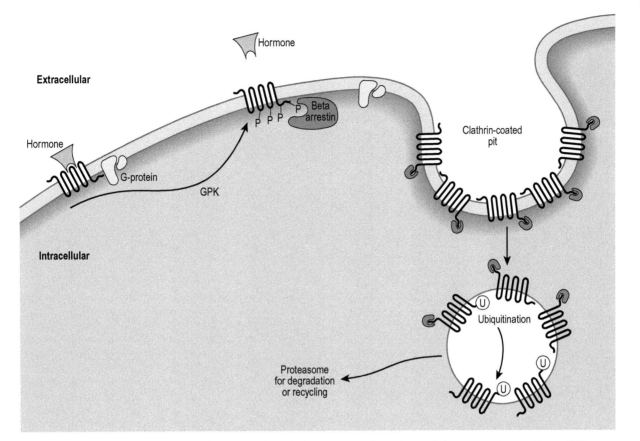

Figure 2.9 Receptor desensitization and internalization. Binding of a hormone to a G-protein coupled receptor attracts a kinase, GPK, which phosphorylates the receptor (P). The phosphorylated receptor attracts beta-arrestin which binds, preventing the receptor from activating G-proteins. Receptors gather in clathrin-coated pits and are internalized, ubiquinated (U) and processed in proteasomes.

which bring about the ubiquitination of both the receptor and the beta arrestin. Ubiquitination is the process of attaching the protein, ubiquitin (so named because it is found in every cell and so is said to be ubiquitous), to the receptor. This has the effect of tagging the receptor for transport to a proteasome where receptors undergo degradation.

Interesting fact

Curiously, although beta arrestins block interactions with G-proteins, they appear to act to enable the receptor to interact with other signalling pathways such as those involving the MAP kinases (see below). This raises the interesting possibility of developing drugs which preferentially facilitate the interaction of the receptor with beta arrestin. For example, a ligand has been developed for the angiotensin II receptor which blocks the G-protein mediated effects (such as raised blood pressure) but specifically stimulates the beta arrestin-mediated effects which include enhanced cell-survival and inhibition of apoptosis (programmed cell death). In cardiovascular disease this would be a most useful drug. It will be interesting to see whether such agents become commonplace in the future.

Receptors which directly activate a protein kinase

The first group of cell-membrane receptors we looked at all act by generating a second messenger which then activates a protein kinase. The other group of cell-surface hormone receptors takes a short-cut by activating a kinase without going through a second messenger. One group of these receptors actually has a protein kinase within the structure of the receptor: this group includes the insulin and growth factor receptors. The second group acts by attracting kinases to the activated receptor: this group includes the growth hormone receptor and cytokine receptors. In both of these receptor groups, dimerization of the receptor is usually an important feature of their activation.

The insulin and growth factor receptor family: receptors with inherent tyrosine kinase activity

This receptor family includes insulin, insulin-like growth factor and a large number of other growth factor receptors (Fig. 2.10). These receptors have a single transmembrane domain, an extracellular ligand binding site and

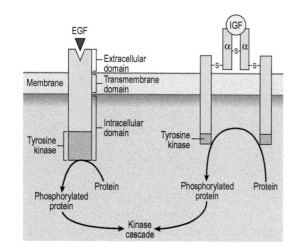

Figure 2.10 Insulin and growth factor receptors. Hormone action through a growth factor receptor, with intrinsic tyrosine kinase activity. The receptor exists in the plasma membrane either as a single transmembrane unit such as the epidermal growth factor (EGF) receptor, or a homodimer such as the insulin or insulin-like growth factor (IGF) receptor. The insulin receptor consists of a dimer with each part having an α and β subunit. The whole receptor is held together by disulphide bridges, indicated as –s– in the diagram. When the hormone binds to the receptor it causes a conformational change within the receptor which activates the protein tyrosine kinase, resulting in the direct phosphorylation of intracellular proteins, and initiation of a kinase cascade.

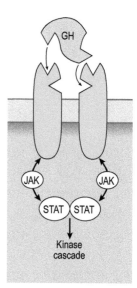

Figure 2.11 Growth hormone and cytokine receptors: Hormone action through a cytokine receptor (or growth hormone, GH receptor). Binding of the hormone to the first receptor causes a conformational change which allows the receptor to dimerize and the hormone to bind to the second receptor subunit; in this case the conformational change in the receptor causes the Janus-associated kinase (JAK) to migrate to the receptor, become activated and phosphorylate signal transducer and activator of transcription (STAT) proteins. JAK was originally called 'Just Another Kinase' but now has the more prosaic name of Janus-associated kinase.

an intracellular tyrosine kinase domain. When the hormone or growth factor binds to the receptor, the conformational change causes two receptors to associate together. This is called receptor dimerization and is an important step in the signalling process for most of these receptors, although the epidermal growth factor receptor (EGF-R) does not appear to form dimers in order to become activated. Dimerization results in activation of the receptor's intrinsic tyrosine kinase activity and phosphorylation of tyrosine residues on target proteins, which include the receptor itself. The phosphorylated receptor attracts a number of accessory proteins which each have the capacity to activate different signalling pathways. All the accessory proteins have a common area called an SH2 domain, which is an area of sequence homology with the src proto-oncogene. This appears to be important for the interaction with the phosphorylated receptor. There is, frankly, a bewildering array of these accessory proteins, with names such as 'son of sevenless' which is known as SOS. The study of these intracellular signalling proteins is worth a book in itself.

The insulin receptor is thought to signal by phosphorylating target proteins called insulin receptor substrate (IRS) proteins. There is a whole family of these proteins which then activate kinase cascades. A large number of proteins are involved in the coordinated cellular response to insulin and growth factor receptor activation.

Interesting fact

As you may have gathered from 'son of sevenless', many of the molecules involved in intracellular signalling systems appear to have been named by post-doctoral researchers with too much time on their hands. The 'death inducing signalling complex' (DISC), for example, includes BIM, BID, BAD, BAK and BAX. BAD is particularly inventive: Bcl-2-associated death promoter. Similarly, as part of the MAPK cascade is MAD/MAX and there is a whole family of 'hedgehog proteins' including, inevitably, Sonic. Sadly, 'Mrs Tiggywinkle' has been renamed shh-b. There is also the SMAD family of transcription factors, activated by transforming growth factor beta signalling: SMAD stands for 'single mothers against decapentaplegic'. Our favourite, though, has to be the Frizzled receptor, activation of which produces Dishevelled.

The growth hormone and cytokine receptors: receptors which attract kinases

These are single-transmembrane domain receptors that do not have inherent kinase activity. After binding of the hormone to one receptor, the receptor dimerizes, apparently via the binding of the same hormone molecule to a second receptor (see Fig. 2.11). The dimerized receptor complex attracts and activates the Janus-associated kinase-signal transducer and activator of transcription (JAK-STAT) pathway (Fig. 2.11). The JAK phosphorylates STAT proteins which then dimerize, move into the nucleus,

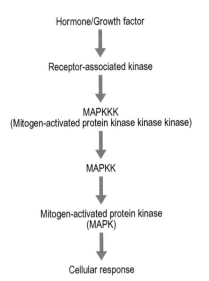

Figure 2.12 The mitogen-activated protein kinase cascade. Each of the kinases in this cascade refers to a family of proteins, which is associated with different aspects of cellular function. For example, the MAPK family includes the kinase P38 which has a role in apoptosis, and ERK1 and ERK2 which have roles in cell growth.

Interesting fact

There is one small family of receptors which falls somewhere between the G-protein coupled receptors and those that directly activate a kinase. The atrial natriuretic peptide family of receptors signals through the generation of cyclic guanosine monophosphate (cGMP). Cyclic GMP is a second messenger like cAMP, produced by the action of an enzyme called guanylyl cyclase. However, the activation of guanylyl cyclase is not mediated by a G-protein. Instead, the receptor itself is a single transmembrane domain protein which possesses intrinsic guanylyl cyclase activity, so cGMP is generated by the receptor itself (Fig. 2.13).

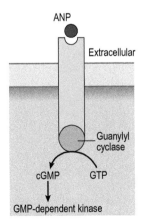

Figure 2.13 Receptor with intrinsic guanylyl cyclase activity. Formation of cGMP leads to activation of kinase pathways and protein phosphorylation. ANP, atrial natriuretic peptide.

bind to specific regulatory elements on gene promoters and so regulate transcription. JAK also phosphorylates the receptor and causes other accessory proteins to associate with the receptor, in a similar manner to the growth factor receptors (above). Again, this results in the activation of a kinase cascade. There are several examples of these, for example the family of mitogen-activated protein kinases (MAPK) which are involved in cell division (Fig. 2.12).

Hormonal regulation of transcription

The effects of all hormones result, at some point, in changes in gene transcription. Hormones that act through kinases all eventually exert effects on the nucleus. In order to achieve this there are regions in the promoter of every hormone-regulated gene that contain 'response elements'. These response elements are consensus sequences of DNA that act as binding sites for specific transcription factors. There is, for example, a cyclic AMP response element (CRE, Fig. 2.14). The protein kinase A, activated by cAMP, translocates to the nucleus and activates a protein called CREB protein which binds to the cAMP response element on the DNA. This attracts CREB binding protein which also binds, activating transcription. Just to complicate matters, there is also a cyclic AMP response element modulator (CREM) which modifies the actions of CREB protein. Proteins such as CREB, which bind to DNA and alter transcription, are called 'transcription factors'. There are many transcription factors in human cells and they regulate the transcription of all genes. From the endocrine point of view, the most important transcription factors are the intracellular hormone receptors.

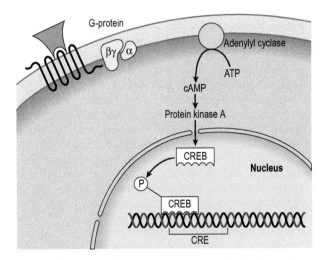

Figure 2.14 Nuclear effects of protein kinase A. Protein kinase A phosphorylates the cyclic AMP response element binding protein (CREB), which then binds to the cyclic AMP response element (CRE) in a gene promoter and initiates transcription.

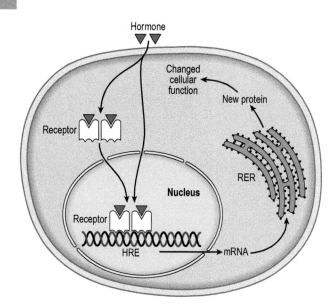

Figure 2.15 Receptors for steroid and thyroid hormones are found inside the cell, in either the cytoplasm or the nucleus. The hormone enters the cell and binds to the receptor. The hormone–receptor complex forms a dimer and binds to hormone response elements (HRE) in the promoter region of certain genes. This can activate or repress transcription of that gene, causing changes in mRNA and therefore new protein formation in the cell. RER is rough endoplasmic reticulum.

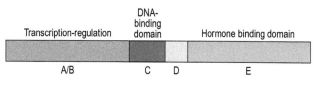

Figure 2.16 Overview of the structure of nuclear receptors.

Intracellular receptors

Steroids, thyroid hormones and calcitriol (active vitamin D), being small and lipophilic, are thought to pass readily across the cell membrane and bind to intracellular receptors, located in the cytoplasm or the nucleus. There is some evidence that these hormones, particularly thyroid hormones, may also be actively transported into the cell. The hormone–receptor complex binds to DNA, to specific response elements in the promoter region of specific genes, and stimulates gene transcription. In this way, steroid and thyroid hormones increase the production of specific proteins and thereby alter cellular function (Fig. 2.15).

The intracellular receptors activated by steroid and other hormones may usefully be considered to be members of the family of transcription factors. Together they are called the nuclear receptor superfamily, comprising 48 members in total. The receptors are structurally closely related although their ligands are diverse. The basic structure of these receptors is shown in Figure 2.16. Each receptor comprises five regions, A, B, C, D and E. AB is a region which is not well-conserved and there is little homology

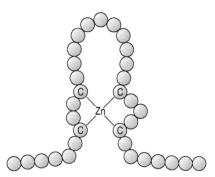

Figure 2.17 A zinc finger motif in a steroid hormone receptor. Each circle represents an amino acid. The 'finger' is stabilized by a zinc atom (Zn) held between cysteine or histidine residues.

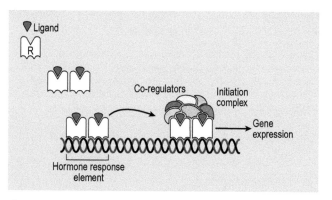

Figure 2.18 Nuclear receptor dimerization and interaction with DNA. In response to ligand binding the receptors dimerize. This can be between two receptors of the same type (homo-dimer) or between two different types of nuclear receptor (hetero-dimer). In both cases the dimer binds to the hormone response element DNA sequence in the gene promoter. The complex attracts co-regulators which can be either co-activators (which permit transcription) or co-repressors (which inhibit transcription). The observation that the same hormone can have different effects in different cells can be explained by the fact that different co-regulators are found in different cells.

between family members. Region C is the DNA binding domain and is highly conserved. It contains two structures called 'zinc fingers' which enable the receptor to bind to specific sites on the DNA. Zinc fingers are given this name because for each 'finger' there is a zinc atom linked to four cysteine residues, which gives this region a stable and characteristic shape (Fig. 2.17). In between the zinc fingers is an area called the P-box which determines the specificity of the receptor for the particular region of DNA. Region E is the hormone binding domain.

The nuclear hormone receptors which we shall be looking at all form dimers when they bind to DNA, although not all transcription factors behave in this way. The dimerized hormone–receptor complex attracts other proteins, co-activators and co-repressors, which together act to regulate gene transcription (Fig. 2.18).

Many drugs act through these nuclear receptors, including the contraceptive pill and anti-diabetic drugs. An understanding of these receptors and how they work is important in understanding drug actions. Mutations in the genes encoding these receptors also gives rise to a number of more rare endocrine disorders, particularly syndromes of hormone resistance: thyroid hormone, vitamin D and androgen resistance. Interestingly, mutations in a nuclear receptor also cause severe insulin insensitivity even though insulin acts through a cell-membrane receptor.

There are two classes of nuclear receptors, class I and class II. We will consider each in turn.

Class I receptors

This receptor subfamily includes all the steroid hormone receptors, but not the calcitriol receptor. There are five types of steroid hormone receptor, corresponding to the five classes of steroid hormone: receptors for glucocorticoid (GR), mineralocorticoid (MR), progesterone (PR), oestrogen (ER) and androgen (AR). These receptors may be located in either the cytoplasm or the nucleus of the target cell and in their resting state, when not bound to a hormone, they are bound to heat shock proteins (HSP), also through the hormone binding domain (Fig. 2.19). In class I receptors, the DNA binding domain of the receptor also contains a region which permits dimerization of the receptors in the presence of DNA. These receptors form only homodimers, which means two receptors of the same type forming a dimer. The receptor only binds to DNA when it is bound to a hormone and it binds to highly specific palindromic (which means reading the same backwards as forwards) regions of the DNA which are called hormone response elements.

Class II receptors

This subfamily of nuclear receptors includes the thyroid hormone receptor and the vitamin D (calcitriol) receptor (Fig. 2.20). The retinoic acid receptor (RXR) and the orphan nuclear receptor called peroxisome proliferator-activated receptor (PPAR gamma) are also included in this group and are significant in the mechanism of action of hormone receptors. The receptors are only located in the nucleus and

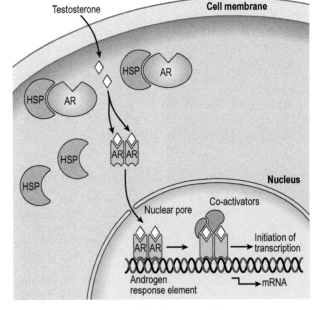

Figure 2.19 Cellular actions of androgens. Androgen receptors are intracellular and in the absence of testosterone they are bound to heat shock protein (HSP) and located in the cytoplasm. In the presence of androgen the HSP dissociates from the receptor allowing the hormone receptor complex to move into the nucleus where it dimerizes with another androgen receptor–hormone complex and binds to the androgen response element on a gene promoter. Various co-activators are attracted to the complex and gene transcription occurs.

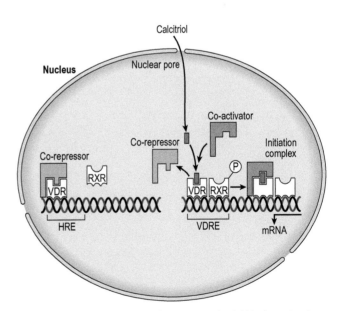

Figure 2.20 Molecular action of calcitriol. Calcitriol binds to vitamin D receptors (VDR) which are located in the nucleus of target cells. Binding of the calcitriol causes the VDR to become phosphorylated which allows it to recruit the retinoic acid receptor (RXR) to form a dimer which binds to the vitamin D response element (VDRE) in a gene promoter. The dimer attracts co-activators to form an initiation complex and permit gene transcription to proceed.

never in the cytoplasm. Class II receptors are able to bind to DNA even in the absence of ligand, and generally bind as heterodimers (two different types of receptors dimerizing: often the hormone receptor dimerizes with RXR). In the absence of ligand, these receptors recruit co-repressors and act to block transcription. When hormone binds to the receptor there is a conformational change in the ligand binding domain so that the co-repressors dissociate and co-activators are recruited. These cause local histone acetylation and transcriptional activation.

Interesting fact

Although the major 'classical' actions of steroids are mediated by nuclear receptors, it is increasingly recognized that steroids can also act through plasma membrane receptors. It is activation of these receptors that accounts for the rapid actions of some steroids, first postulated by Hans Selye in the 1940s, when it was shown that certain steroids can act as anaesthetics. These steroids act so quickly, within a few seconds, that their actions cannot possibly be mediated by a genomic mechanism.

Disorders of receptor function

There are some well-characterized clinical conditions which arise from mutations of the genes encoding different receptors: Laron syndrome, for example, where there is a defect in the growth hormone receptor. In general, receptor gene mutations cause varying degrees of loss of function of the receptor. Where there is a significant loss of function in a developmentally significant receptor this usually causes spontaneous abortion of the foetus. In some cases we have learned a great deal about the normal functioning of a receptor system from examples of gene mutations causing changes in function. Several clinical conditions resulting from receptor defects are described in the following chapters, but these generally do not involve G-protein coupled receptors (GPCR). Despite the complexity of the GPCR system, receptor defects are very rare. The most commonly cited examples of G protein receptor mutations are those which result in constitutive activity of the receptor, which means that the receptor is able to activate signalling pathways even when no ligand is present. Spontaneous mutations of the thyroid stimulating hormone (TSH) receptor produce a constitutively active receptor leading to the development of highly active ('hot') thyroid nodules which secrete excess thyroid hormone. There is also an hereditary disorder of a constitutively active luteinizing hormone (LH) receptor which causes precocious puberty in males.

THE HYPOTHALAMUS AND PITUITARY PART I:
THE HYPOTHALAMUS AND POSTERIOR PITUITARY

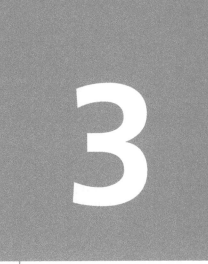

Chapter objectives

After studying this chapter you should be able to:

1. Describe the locations of the hypothalamus and pituitary and explain how they are connected, both anatomically and physiologically.

2. Describe the hormones secreted from the posterior pituitary and outline their actions.

3. Describe how these hormones are synthesized and secreted.

4. Explain what is meant by the term 'neuroendocrine reflex'.

5. Describe the clinical effects of under-production of arginine vasopressin.

6. Explain the science underlying the clinical tests used to diagnose this disorder.

Introduction

The hypothalamus and pituitary gland are the principal organizers of the endocrine system. The hypothalamus is part of the brain and is directly connected to the pituitary gland. The hypothalamus receives a wide range of neural inputs that can alter its secretory functions in response to conditions such as stress, exercise and even the time of day. It is subject to negative feedback regulation by both pituitary and target organ hormones. Because of this complex set of inputs and outputs, the hypothalamus acts to integrate many hormonal and neural responses (Fig. 3.1).

The pituitary has two quite distinct parts: the posterior pituitary, which is an extension of nerve cells from the hypothalamus; and the anterior pituitary, which is linked by blood vessels to the hypothalamus. The hypothalamus controls the function of both the anterior and posterior pituitary, but achieves this in different ways. The hormones secreted by the posterior pituitary are synthesized in nerve cells in the hypothalamus and transported along nerve axons to the posterior pituitary, from which they are simply released from the nerve terminals. However, the hypothalamus also produces a range of hormones that act on the different cell types of the anterior pituitary to control their secretory activity. These releasing and inhibitory hormones travel from the hypothalamus to the anterior pituitary in a network of blood vessels called a portal circulation.

Interesting fact

The parts of the pituitary gland have been called by different names at different times: posterior pituitary is the same as the neurohypophysis; anterior pituitary is the same as the adenohypophysis.

The word 'pituitary' derives from the wonderfully onomatopoeic Greek word *ptuo* (to spit), hence the Latin *pituita* (mucus). This is because it was once thought that the function of the pituitary was to allow mucus produced by the brain to drain down the nose!

Where can i find the hypothalamus and pituitary?

As its name implies, the hypothalamus is located beneath the thalamus at the base of the brain. The hypothalamus is closely related to the optic chiasm (inferiorly), mamillary bodies (posteriorly) and the third ventricle (superiorly) (Fig. 3.2).

The hypothalamus is a part of the brain that acts as a control centre for a range of diverse processes, including regulation of the autonomic nervous system, body temperature, water balance, appetite and mood. It does this by integrating monitoring processes with regulatory systems, and neural processes with endocrine systems. For example, the hypothalamus contains cells that produce the anti-diuretic hormone, arginine vasopressin, cells that monitor the concentration of plasma (osmoreceptors), and an area that regulates thirst, all connected

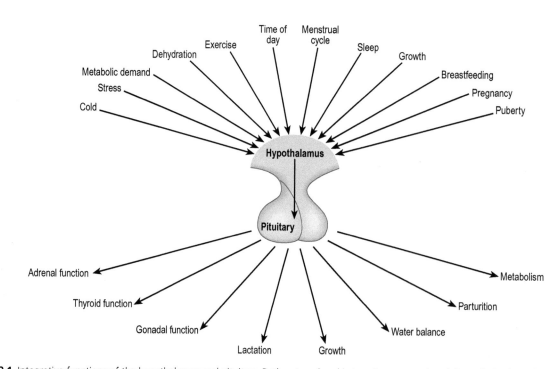

Figure 3.1 Integrative functions of the hypothalamus and pituitary. Both external and internal cues are relayed through the hypothalamus, leading to hormone secretion from the pituitary. The pituitary hormones regulate a number of important physiological processes.

Hypothalamic tumour: 1

Case history

Mr Jones, a 30-year-old man, began passing a lot of urine approximately 6 weeks earlier. He needed to pass urine once or twice per hour and was woken from his sleep by a full bladder at least four or five times during the night. He felt unusually thirsty, was constantly drinking water and had noticed that his urine was very pale. In recent weeks, he had been having headaches at night and on waking. His libido had decreased over recent months and he had problems maintaining an erection. Most recently, he had become very forgetful.

The medical history was unremarkable. Mr Jones lived with his girlfriend and they had no children. He worked as an engineer.

He had been to see his GP, who had tested his urine and found no protein or glucose present. The GP also found no abnormalities in Mr Jones' blood glucose or calcium levels. At this stage, the GP referred Mr Jones to an endocrine clinic.

On examination in the clinic, he looked uncomfortable and dehydrated with a dry mouth and tongue. His temperature was normal, 37°C, but the resting pulse rate was 100 b.p.m., with a blood pressure of 105/65 mmHg. Fundoscopy revealed the optic nerve to be swollen in both eyes. Testing of the visual fields showed a loss of vision in both temporal (outer) halves of the field (see Fig. 3.3). He was confused and could not remember how he had got to the hospital or what he had eaten that day, but he knew the name of his girlfriend and could remember distant events.

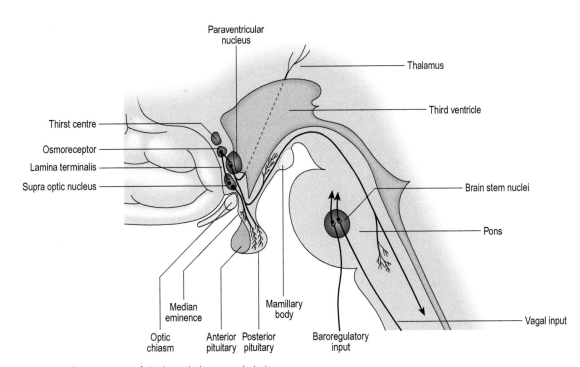

Figure 3.2 Diagram of the location of the hypothalamus and pituitary.

by a neural network. The areas of the hypothalamus that are anatomically or functionally distinct are known as nuclei. Several of the hypothalamic nuclei have primarily endocrine functions, most notably the paraventricular nucleus, but also the supraoptic and ventromedial nuclei. These are located in the region of the hypothalamus close to the third ventricle.

The hypothalamus is physically connected to the pituitary gland by the pituitary stalk. The pituitary gland is located in the pituitary fossa, which is a hollow in the sphenoid bone at the base of the brain (Fig. 3.2). The pituitary lies outside the blood–brain barrier and is not considered to be a part of the brain. Anatomically, the pituitary gland is very close to the optic chiasm and large pituitary tumours often cause visual disturbances (Fig. 3.3). The normal pituitary gland weighs less than 1 g and is approximately 14 mm across, although it increases in size during pregnancy and shrinks with age.

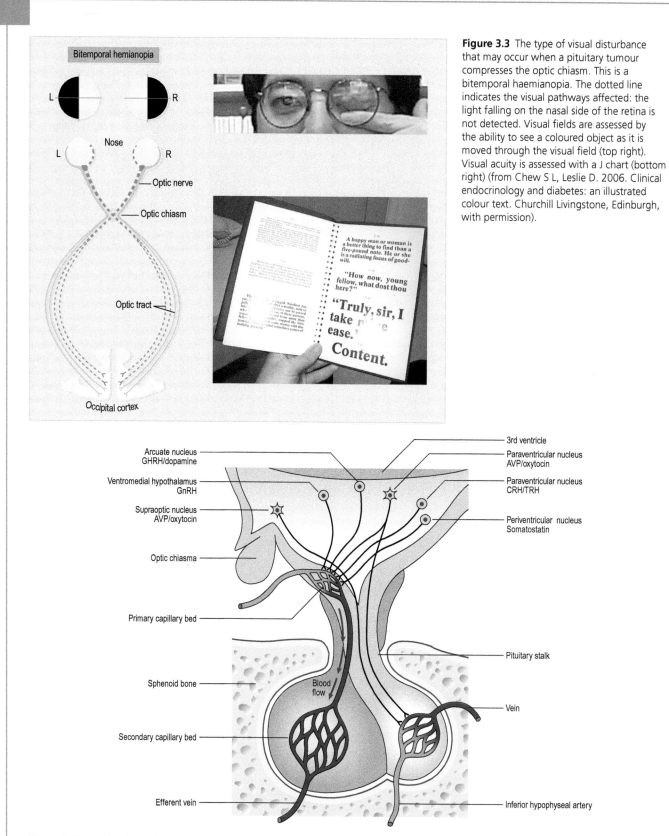

Figure 3.3 The type of visual disturbance that may occur when a pituitary tumour compresses the optic chiasm. This is a bitemporal haemianopia. The dotted line indicates the visual pathways affected: the light falling on the nasal side of the retina is not detected. Visual fields are assessed by the ability to see a coloured object as it is moved through the visual field (top right). Visual acuity is assessed with a J chart (bottom right) (from Chew S L, Leslie D. 2006. Clinical endocrinology and diabetes: an illustrated colour text. Churchill Livingstone, Edinburgh, with permission).

Figure 3.4 Neural and vascular connections between the hypothalamus and pituitary. The hypothalamus and posterior pituitary have a direct neural link, whereas the anterior pituitary has a vascular connection to the hypothalamus. Note the separate blood supply to the two parts of the pituitary. Disruption of the portal system results in failure of anterior pituitary hormone secretion, but usually not of posterior pituitary hormones. The neurons with star-shaped cell bodies are magnocellular neurons and the round cell bodies indicate parvocellular neurons. AVP, arginine vasopressin; CRH, corticotropin releasing hormone; GnRH, gonadotropin releasing hormone; PVN, paraventricular nucleus; TRH, thyrotropin releasing hormone.

Interesting fact

The pituitary fossa is also known as the sella turcica, due to its apparent resemblance to a Turkish style of saddle. More bizarrely, 'hypothalamus' comes from the Greek for 'under the bed'!

Connection between the hypothalamus and pituitary

The pituitary stalk, which connects the hypothalamus to the pituitary gland, carries both blood vessels and nerve fibres. The anterior pituitary is connected to the hypothalamus by a vascular connection through the hypophyseal portal system. A portal system is a vascular connection with two sets of capillary beds. The first set of capillaries is in the hypothalamus and blood passes through the portal veins in the pituitary stalk to the second set of capillaries in the anterior pituitary (Fig. 3.4). In this way, agents released from the hypothalamus can be delivered to the pituitary where they act on pituitary cells to control hormone synthesis and release.

The posterior pituitary consists of fibres of the magnocellular and parvocellular neurons, which carry the posterior pituitary hormones from the hypothalamus.

Development of the hypothalamus and pituitary

The posterior pituitary is neural in origin and, together with the pituitary stalk, derives from a down-growth of the diencephalon. The anterior pituitary is ectodermal and derives from Rathke's pouch, an outgrowth of the buccal cavity. The two tissues migrate to lie adjacent to each other and form the pituitary gland. The anterior component is larger than the posterior part, comprising about two-thirds of the gland.

The hormones of the hypothalamus

We have already seen that the hypothalamus is connected to the pituitary gland in two different ways: by a portal vascular system to the anterior pituitary and by a direct neural connection to the posterior pituitary. So it is not surprising that the hypothalamus produces hormones that are released into the portal blood system to act on the anterior pituitary and other hormones which pass directly down the nerve connection and are released from the posterior pituitary. We will learn more about the hormones which act on the anterior pituitary in the next chapter. These hormones are a mix of 'releasing hormones' and 'release-inhibiting hormones' (see Table 4.2). Their concerted action is critical in the regulation of anterior pituitary function.

Case 3.1 Hypothalamic tumour: 2

Case note: Investigation

Given the combination of abnormal regulation of water balance and visual disturbance, can you localize the problem area?

The main site of control of water excretion is the hypothalamus, which contains both osmoreceptors and cells that produce the anti-diuretic hormone, vasopressin. A homonymous bitemporal hemianopia is characteristic of lesions of the optic chiasm. So the combination of these two features would suggest a lesion affecting both the hypothalamus and the optic chiasm.

What further tests would you want to carry out?

Blood and urine tests were performed and showed serum levels of sodium, 154 mmol/L; serum urea, 15 mmol/L; plasma glucose, 8.2 mmol/L; urine osmolality, 50 mOsm/kg and serum osmolality, 295 mOsm/kg.

An MRI scan was performed and showed a large tumour of the hypothalamus with pressure or infiltration of the surrounding structures (Fig. 3.5).

Psychometric testing by a psychologist would be helpful as a baseline to quantify the extent of Mr Jones' short-term memory problem.

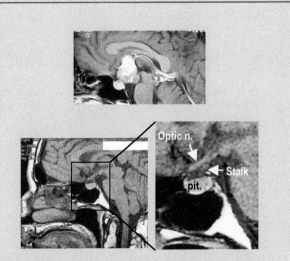

Figure 3.5 Magnetic resonance images of the pituitary gland and hypothalamus in the sagittal plane. The top image shows the tumour destroying Mr Jones' hypothalamus. The irregular tumour contains many blood vessels and shows a bright signal after contrast injection. The lower image shows a normal pituitary and hypothalamic anatomy. Chew S. and Leslie D. Clinical Endocrinology and Diabetes: an illustrated colour text. Churchill Livingstone, Edinburgh.

The hormones of the posterior pituitary

The posterior pituitary secretes two hormones, oxytocin and vasopressin. Vasopressin is also called arginine vasopressin (AVP) or sometimes anti-diuretic hormone (ADH) because of its major physiological action. Both oxytocin and arginine vasopressin are small peptides, of only nine amino acids, seven of which are common to both (Fig. 3.6). They are synthesized in the hypothalamus, in the magnocellular neurons of the supra-optic and paraventricular nuclei (Fig. 3.4). Different subsets of the neurons produce either oxytocin or arginine vasopressin. They are both made as part of a large precursor peptide called neurophysin, which is processed into the mature peptide hormones as it passes along the neural tract. These hormones are transported down the nerve axons

Arginine vasopressin

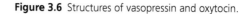

Cys–Tyr–Phe–Gln–Asn–Cys–Pro–Arg–Gly–NH₂

Oxytocin

Cys–Tyr–Ile–Gln–Asn–Cys–Pro–Leu–Gly–NH₂

Figure 3.6 Structures of vasopressin and oxytocin.

in the supraoptic–hypothalamic tract into the posterior pituitary. Release of oxytocin or arginine vasopressin is brought about by an action potential in the nerve.

Interesting fact

The vasopressin/oxytocin family of peptide hormones provides one of the best examples of peptide evolution (Fig. 3.7). Peptides related to vasopressin/oxytocin are found in all animal species, from hydra, to worms and snails, to fishes, birds and mammals. In vertebrates, the ancestor for both peptides is thought to be vasotocin, a peptide still found in the hagfish and lamprey, primitive jawless fish which originated over 500 million years ago.

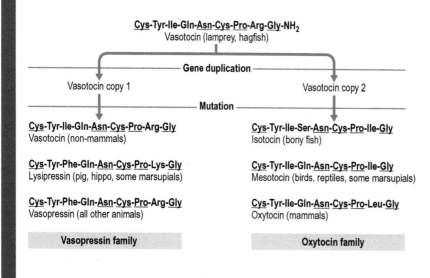

Figure 3.7 Evolution of oxytocin and vasopressin. Underlining shows where an amino acid occurs in the same place in all members of the hormone family. In this family there is a high degree of conservancy as five of the eight amino acids are common to all the hormones.

The accepted mechanism for peptide evolution is gene duplication, where a section of chromosome is duplicated in one copy and deleted from the other at cell division. Mutations occurring in the duplicated gene can then produce a new functional peptide or protein without losing the original function which is continued by the intact first copy of the gene.

Duplication of the vasotocin gene in primitive jawless fish about 500 million years ago is thought to have given rise to the vasopressin/oxytocin family of peptides which are found in pairs (one form of oxytocin and one form of vasopressin) throughout all vertebrates (Fig. 3.7).

Release of posterior pituitary hormones is part of a neuroendocrine reflex: oxytocin secretion and actions

A neuroendocrine reflex involves the release of a hormone from a nerve terminal in response to depolarization of the nerve (Fig. 3.8). It differs from simple neurotransmission because the hormone is released into the blood, rather than a synaptic cleft. The control of oxytocin release makes a good illustration of the principles of a neuroendocrine reflex. This hormone has a role in both parturition (childbirth) and lactation. It does not influence the production of milk, but is essential for the release of

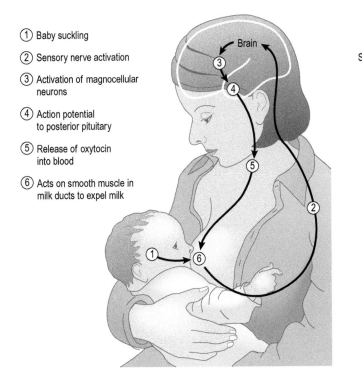

① Baby suckling

② Sensory nerve activation

③ Activation of magnocellular neurons

④ Action potential to posterior pituitary

⑤ Release of oxytocin into blood

⑥ Acts on smooth muscle in milk ducts to expel milk

Figure 3.8 Neuroendocrine reflex. Suckling of the baby causes a sensory nerve signal to be sent to the brain. The signal is relayed to the hypothalamus where activation of magnocellular neurons causes release of the hormone oxytocin from the posterior pituitary. Oxytocin travels in blood and acts on the primed breast ducts, causing smooth muscle contraction and milk expulsion.

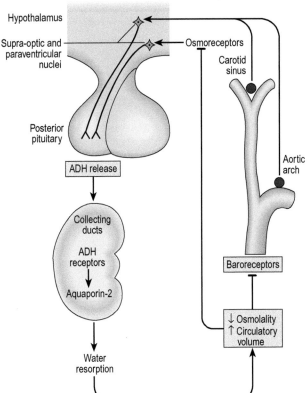

Figure 3.9 Regulation and action of vasopressin (ADH, anti-diuretic hormone). This is another example of a neuroendocrine reflex: the baroreceptors in the aortic arch and carotid sinus send neural signals to the hypothalamus, resulting in the release of a hormone, ADH (from Chew S L, Leslie D. 2006. Clinical endocrinology and diabetes: an illustrated colour text. Churchill Livingstone, Edinburgh, with permission).

milk: the milk ejection reflex. During lactation, suckling initiates a neural signal from the nipple to the brain. This signal is relayed to the hypothalamus and an action potential is sent along the neural tract to the posterior pituitary, causing the release of oxytocin from the posterior pituitary into the bloodstream. The oxytocin acts on the smooth muscle surrounding the alveoli in the breast, causing contraction of the muscle and ejection of milk from the nipple.

Recently, there have been significant advances in our understanding of the actions of oxytocin. It has been known for many years that oxytocin plays a significant role in social behaviour in many animals. Recently, considerable attention has been given to the role of oxytocin in social bonding in humans. It has been suggested that maternal oxytocin levels before and after birth correlate with the strength of the mother–infant bond and that oxytocin released during sexual intercourse increases the bond between sexual partners. Other complex behaviours which appear to be affected by oxytocin include a person's level of trust and generosity.

Therapeutically, oxytocin is used as a labour-inducing drug, to increase uterine contractions and also to reduce postpartum bleeding. It is perhaps worth noting that there are no recognized clinical conditions of oxytocin excess or insufficiency.

Regulation of vasopressin secretion

Like oxytocin, arginine vasopressin release is part of a neuroendocrine reflex. The major stimulus to the release of arginine vasopressin is an increase in plasma osmolality (Box 3.1), which is detected by osmoreceptors in the hypothalamus (Fig. 3.9). A neural signal is relayed to the paraventricular and supraoptic nuclei and an action potential is generated in the nerves supplying the posterior pituitary, causing the release of arginine vasopressin into the blood. A decrease in either blood volume or blood pressure also stimulates the release of arginine vasopressin. A fall in blood volume is detected by the baroreceptors in the left atrium of the heart, whereas a decreased blood pressure is detected by the baroreceptors in the aortic arch and carotid artery. However, the most important factor in regulating arginine vasopressin secretion is plasma osmolality, with a normal threshold of 280 mmol/kg. This threshold is slightly lower in pregnancy and significantly reduced by a fall in blood volume.

Box 3.1 What is plasma osmolality?

The amount of osmotically active particles in a biological fluid is expressed in osmoles. Technically, the osmolality is the number of osmoles per kilogram of solvent (plasma or urine) and is the primary measure of concentration. The very similar term 'osmolarity' refers to the number of osmoles per *litre* of solvent. As 1 L of water weighs 1 kg, these two terms tend to be used interchangeably. More than 90% of the solute in plasma is sodium and its associated anions, chloride and bicarbonate. Glucose and urea make up most of the remaining solutes. The concentration of solute determines the freezing point of a liquid and this is how osmolality is measured in the laboratory. The osmolality of plasma can also be estimated by the formula:

Osmolality (mOsm/L) = 2 × sodium (mmol/L) + glucose (mmol/L) + urea (mmol/L).

Table 3.1 Actions of arginine vasopressin (anti-diuretic hormone)

Tissue	Receptor subtype	Effect
Kidney	V_2 receptor	Anti-diuresis (by increasing water reabsorption)
Pituitary gland (corticotroph cells)	V_{1b} receptor	Stimulates release of ACTH (acts with CRH)
Vascular smooth muscle	V_{1a} receptor	Causes vasoconstriction
Vascular endothelial cells	V_2 receptor	Release of clotting factors

Actions of arginine vasopressin

The actions of arginine vasopressin are summarised in (Table 3.1). Arginine vasopressin is a short-acting hormone, with a plasma half-life of around 15 min. Its main site of action is the collecting duct of the kidney, where it increases water resorption. This has the effect of reducing the urine volume and explains the alternative name for arginine vasopressin of 'anti-diuretic hormone' (ADH), as diuresis is the formation of urine.

Arginine vasopressin increases water resorption by making the renal collecting ducts more permeable to water (Fig. 3.9). It achieves this by binding to the V_2 subclass of receptors on the basolateral surface of cells lining the renal collecting ducts. The effect of activating these vasopressin receptors is to stimulate production of a protein called aquaporin 2 on the apical membrane of these cells (Fig. 3.10). Aquaporin 2 forms an open channel that allows water to pass out of the lumen of the collecting duct. The physiological effect of arginine vasopressin

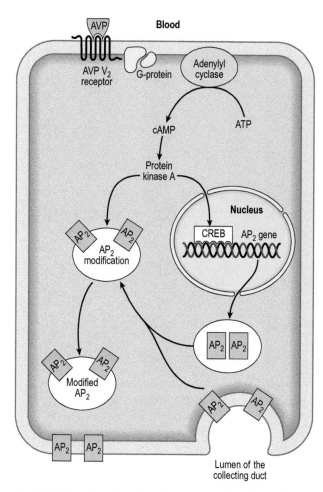

Figure 3.10 Cellular action of arginine vasopressin on the collecting duct. Arginine vasopressin (AVP) binds to specific V_2 receptors on the surface of the collecting duct cell. The V_2 receptor is coupled via a G-protein, to adenylyl cyclase and activation of the receptor causes an increase in cAMP, which activates protein kinase A. This has two main effects, firstly to increase the transcription of the gene encoding the water transporter protein aquaporin 2 (AP_2). Protein kinase A also increases the recycling of the internalized aquaporin 2 proteins and causes more AP_2 to be present on the luminal surface of the cell. This has the effect of increasing water uptake from the lumen of the collecting duct.

is the conservation of water in the body by causing the production of smaller volumes of more highly concentrated urine, which may be more than twice the osmolality of plasma (Fig. 3.11). Arginine vasopressin is not the only hormone involved in regulating blood volume and osmolality: an overview of the integrated control of blood pressure, volume and osmolality is given in Chapter 13.

As its name implies, arginine vasopressin also has actions on the vascular system, causing increases in blood pressure through the activation of vasopressin V_1 receptors in blood vessels. The vasopressin receptors in the kidney (called V_2) are slightly different from those in blood vessels (called V_1). This is exploited in the development of drugs that bind preferentially to V_2 receptors

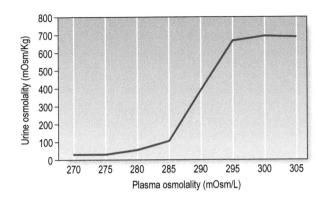

Figure 3.11 Effects of vasopressin on the kidney: the relationship between plasma and urine osmolalities. As plasma osmolality increases, the actions of AVP (ADH) cause an increase in urine osmolality until a plateau is reached (from Chew S L, Leslie D. 2006. Clinical endocrinology and diabetes: an illustrated colour text. Churchill Livingstone, Edinburgh, with permission).

and so can be used to treat diabetes insipidus without adverse effects on blood pressure.

Arginine vasopressin also has a completely different role as a hypothalamic releasing factor. It acts together with corticotropin releasing hormone to stimulate the release of corticotropin from the anterior pituitary gland. This is a synergistic effect, with the effects of corticotropin releasing hormone and arginine vasopressin acting together being significantly greater than either acting alone (see Ch. 6).

Clinically, AVP is used as replacement therapy, to treat the disorder of diabetes insipidus. It is also used to reduce bleeding during gastrointestinal surgery, making use of its vasoconstrictor properties. Injections of AVP are also used to boost factor VIII concentrations in mild haemophilia.

Interesting fact

Most peptide hormones have to be administered by injection. However, desmopressin, the synthetic analogue of arginine vasopressin, can be administered orally in tablet form, or by nasal spray. However, there is a difference in the dose required depending on the route of administration: given orally the effective dose is 100 mg, by nasal spray it is 10–20 mg, but when administered by subcutaneous injection only 1 mg is required.

Disorders of vasopressin secretion and action

Deficiency

A deficiency of arginine vasopressin secretion or action results in a condition termed diabetes insipidus. Diabetes

Case 3.1 Hypothalamic tumour: 3

Case note: Explanation of symptoms and signs

When vasopressin secretion is damaged, as in Mr Jones' case, aquaporin 2 no longer forms a water channel for reabsorption of water, and water loss in the urine results in large volumes of dilute urine. Thirst and excessive drinking are caused by a high concentration of plasma, due to water losses in the urine. This condition is called diabetes insipidus. The consequent dehydration results in decreased blood volume with increased pulse rate and hypotension.

The visual impairment is due to compression of the optic chiasm, resulting in optic neuritis and homonymous bitemporal hemianopia. The loss of short-term memory is due to damage to the mamillary bodies. Both of these effects are due to space-occupying effects of the tumour on adjacent structures.

The headaches on waking are a classical symptom of an intracranial mass, which causes stretching of the dura mater.

Impaired sexual function can result from any disease of the pituitary or hypothalamus that impairs gonadotropin production.

insipidus is called 'hypothalamic' or 'cranial' when there is a failure of arginine vasopressin secretion, and 'nephrogenic' when there is renal insensitivity to the actions of arginine vasopressin ('vasopressin resistance'). The two conditions are easily distinguished by giving the patient desmopressin and testing the response of urine concentration. In cranial diabetes insipidus, the urine becomes very concentrated (i.e. the urine volume drops and urine osmolality rises). Conversely, in nephrogenic diabetes insipidus, the urine does not change in response to desmopressin administration.

Diabetes insipidus is characterized by polyuria, the production of large volumes of very dilute urine, accompanied by polydipsia, excessive thirst. There is no single cause of either hypothalamic or nephrogenic diabetes insipidus: neither is a common disorder. However, the hypothalamic form may be caused by a tumour, or may result from trauma to the brain. It may be caused by surgery to adjacent areas, such as the pituitary gland, and in these cases, the disorder is often transient. Hypothalamic diabetes insipidus is treated by administration of a synthetic analogue of vasopressin, termed desmopressin, which has all the renal effects of vasopressin but has less effect on the vasculature because of much weaker binding to V_1 vasopressin receptors.

Nephrogenic diabetes insipidus occasionally results from a genetic defect in vasopressin receptors, although this is rare. More commonly, it is a result of metabolic disturbances, such as hypercalcaemia, or seen as an adverse drug reaction. It is a recognized complication of lithium therapy, which is used to treat bipolar disorder. Nephrogenic diabetes insipidus is usually treated by

THE HYPOTHALAMUS AND POSTERIOR PITUITARY

3

THE ENDOCRINE SYSTEM | 35

correcting the underlying metabolic problem or discontinuing drug therapy. However, it may also be treated with drugs that increase renal sensitivity to arginine vasopressin, such as chlorpropamide.

Other causes of polyuria, polydipsia and thirst include diabetes mellitus (distinguished by abnormally high blood sugar levels) and primary polydipsia. There are several causes of primary polydipsia, including psychogenic (where patients with mental illness drink 10 L of water per day) and idiopathic (where otherwise healthy people have a lowered osmotic threshold for thirst). Primary polydipsia can usually be distinguished from diabetes insipidus by the fact that the plasma is dilute, rather than concentrated. A water deprivation test may also be useful: in primary polydipsia the urine becomes appropriately concentrated on dehydration; in hypothalamic diabetes insipidus the urine becomes appropriately concentrated only after desmopressin is given, and in nephrogenic diabetes insipidus the urine osmolality does not change with either dehydration or desmopressin.

Interesting fact

Before the advent of modern methods of urine analysis, the only way to test urine was for the physician to dip their finger into a sample and taste it. This is how the two types of diabetes got their names: in diabetes mellitus (a disorder of glucose metabolism) the urine characteristically tastes sweet, whereas in diabetes insipidus (a disorder of water metabolism) the urine was considered to 'lack flavour'.

Excess arginine vasopressin secretion

Excess vasopressin secretion results in the syndrome of inappropriate anti-diuretic hormone (SIADH), where the

---

Case 3.1   Hypothalamic tumour: 4

Case note: Management
How can treatment be guided by physiological principles?

The first principle of treatment is to prevent dehydration by ensuring an adequate water intake. The second is to replace arginine vasopressin with a synthetic analogue called desmopressin. Desmopressin acts like arginine vasopressin and reduces urinary water excretion and increases urine osmolality. Finally, the underlying disease process must be treated by surgical removal of the tumour, although destruction of the hypothalamic nuclei may leave permanent diabetes insipidus. The damage that has been caused to adjacent structures is also likely to be irreversible, leaving Mr Jones with permanent disability.

Case 3.1   Hypothalamic tumour: 5

A suggested exercise

Estimate Mr Jones' plasma osmolality: sodium concentration 154 mmol/L, urea 15 mmol/L and glucose 8 mmol/L.

(Answer: $[2 \times 154] + 15 + 8 = 331$ mOsm/L).

The osmolality of Mr Jones' urine was <50 mOsm/kg. What would it be if he did not have diabetes insipidus and his serum osmolality was 331 mOsm/L?

(Answer: It should be $>2 \times 331 = 662$ mOsm/kg).

---

water retention has such a diluting effect on plasma that it results in low plasma sodium levels (hyponatraemia) with a normal plasma volume. The syndrome is called 'inappropriate ADH secretion' because the appropriate physiological response would be to reduce AVP (ADH) secretion and increase diuresis. The problem in SIADH is that the AVP levels are inappropriately high.

In SIADH, the urine is usually more concentrated, i.e. has a higher osmolality, than plasma. The symptoms of SIADH are essentially those of hyponatraemia, with headache, nausea, vomiting, confusion and ultimately coma. SIADH has many causes including neoplasms such as lung cancer (which can secrete vasopressin), neurological disorders such as meningitis, lung disease such as pneumonia and tuberculosis, and prescribed drugs such as carbamazepine. Tubercular lung tissue has been shown to contain measureable amounts of arginine vasopressin, as have some forms of lung cancer. In pneumonia it is not clear whether the infection causes local secretion of arginine vasopressin in the lung or whether it affects hypothalamic production.

Thirst

If you look at Figure 3.1, the connection between dehydration acting on the hypothalamus and, as a result, the pituitary acting to regulate water balance, is thirst. Thirst is such a common experience that we assume it is a simple process, but the regulation of thirst is very complex, involving angiotensin II, arginine vasopressin and central and peripheral receptors. For a summary of the hormonal control of blood pressure, osmolality and thirst, see Chapter 13.

Water intoxication occurs when an individual drinks more fluids than they can handle in a physiologically appropriate manner. It can have many causes, including the psychogenic polydipsia associated with schizophrenia, and the excessive drinking seen following ingestion of Ecstasy (MDMA), which usually occurs in a misguided attempt to avoid dehydration and hyperthermia.

Other hypothalamic hormones

In addition to oxytocin and vasopressin, the hypothalamus produces two neuropeptide hormones called the orexins, also known as hypocretins. These hormones, orexin A and orexin B, have about 50% homology. Orexin A has 33 amino acids while orexin B has 28. They are released from cells in the lateral and posterior hypothalamus and have effects on both wakefulness and eating. Orexin promotes wakefulness and disorders of orexin production are thought to be associated with the sleep disorder, narcolepsy. Orexin also stimulates hunger. Its secretion is inhibited by glucose and by leptin, an appetite regulating hormone (see Ch. 13). Pharmacologically, orexin agonists have been proposed as a possible treatment for narcolepsy and also in the treatment of addictive disorders.

THE HYPOTHALAMUS AND PITUITARY PART II:
THE ANTERIOR PITUITARY

4

Chapter objectives

After studying this chapter you should be able to:

1. Describe the structure of the anterior pituitary and the hormones produced by each cell type.

2. Describe how the secretion of each anterior pituitary hormone is regulated.

3. Describe the physiological effects of each anterior pituitary hormone.

4. Describe the effects of under- and over-production of growth hormone.

5. Describe the regulation and actions of prolactin.

6. Explain the science underlying the clinical tests used to diagnose disorders of growth hormone secretion.

Introduction

In the previous chapter, we looked at the structure and location of the pituitary gland, and its relationship to the hypothalamus. We saw that the anterior pituitary is linked to the hypothalamus by a portal blood system in which the blood flows from the primary capillary plexus in the hypothalamus to the secondary capillary plexus in the anterior pituitary. This portal system carries hormones from the hypothalamus to the anterior pituitary and is key to understanding the functions of the anterior pituitary. One of the main functions of the anterior pituitary is to secrete hormones that control the activity of other endocrine glands, particularly the gonads, thyroid and adrenal. So it can be seen that the hypothalamus and pituitary are the master controllers of several completely independent endocrine systems, such as the hypothalamo–pituitary–adrenal axis (HPA axis) and the hypothalamo–pituitary–gonadal axis. When considering the anterior pituitary, the four 'tropic hormones' are often considered separately. The tropic hormones are those hormones that regulate other endocrine glands: LH, FSH, ACTH and TSH. The regulation of these hormones will be considered in detail in Chapters 6–9. In this chapter, we will focus on prolactin and growth hormone. It is worth noting at an early stage that the actions of growth hormone should be considered alongside the actions of a growth factor, called insulin-like growth factor-1 (IGF-1). This is because growth hormone exerts many of its actions indirectly, through the production of IGF-1 by liver and bone.

Structure of the anterior pituitary

The anterior pituitary is composed of five different cell types, each of which secretes a different hormone (Table 4.1). The most abundant type of secretory cell in the anterior pituitary is the somatotroph. These cells account for around 50% of the secretory cells in the gland and are principally located in the anterior wings of the gland. Lactotrophs are located throughout the gland and represent between 10% and 30% of the secretory cells. These

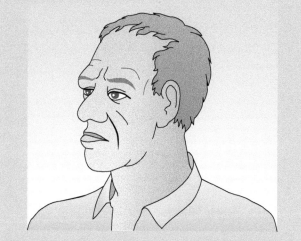
Table 4.1 Major cell types of the anterior pituitary and the hormones they secrete

Cell type	Hormone	Structure	Size
Acidophil cells			
Somatotrophs	Growth hormone	Protein	≈22 000 Da; 191 amino acids
Lactotrophs	Prolactin	Protein	≈23 000 Da; 199 amino acids
Basophil cells			
Thyrotrophs	TSH	Glycoprotein	≈30 000 Da
Gonadotrophs	LH and FSH	Glycoprotein	≈25 000 Da
Corticotrophs	ACTH	Peptide	39 amino acids

two cell types are described as acidophils because they stain with acidic dyes. The other cell types are basophils because they stain with basic dyes. There are three types of basophils, the most numerous being gonadotrophs which make up about 20% of the secretory cells in the gland, with corticotrophs 10% and thyrotrophs 5%. The basophils are mostly found in the medial section of the anterior pituitary. All the secretory cells of the anterior pituitary contain secretory granules and are histologically typical of peptide-secreting cells (see Ch. 1). There is another group of cells, called folliculostellate cells, in the anterior pituitary which make up around 10% of the gland volume and are distributed throughout the gland. These cells do not contain secretory granules and do not stain with either acid or basic dyes. Their function is not clear but it is possible that they are pituitary stem cells, capable of differentiating into one of the secretory cell types.

The hormones of the anterior pituitary

The hormones of the anterior pituitary are all peptides (Fig. 4.2). Prolactin (Prl) and growth hormone (GH) are large single-chain polypeptides. Luteinizing hormone (LH), follicle stimulating hormone (FSH) and thyroid stimulating hormone (TSH) are members of a family of large double-chained glycoproteins that also includes human chorionic gonadotropin (hCG). These hormones consist of two glycosylated polypeptide chains linked by disulphide bridges. The α-subunit is identical for all members of this hormone family and it is the hormone-specific β-subunit that distinguishes these hormones. Adrenocorticotropic hormone (ACTH) is relatively small, comprising just 39 amino acids, but it is synthesized as part of a much larger precursor protein, termed pro-opiomelanocortin (POMC), which also gives rise to β-endorphin and the opioid peptides met- and leu-enkephalin (Fig. 4.3).

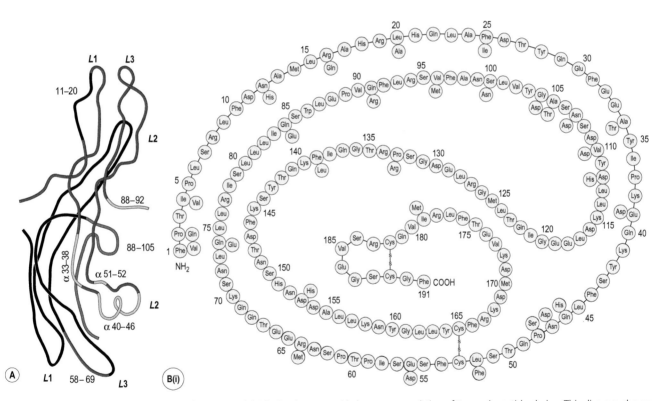

Figure 4.2 Structures of anterior pituitary hormones. (A) TSH is a large peptide hormone consisting of two polypeptide chains. This diagram shows the tertiary structure of TSH. The α-chain is shown as a grey line and the β-chain as a black line. The folding of the peptides, producing the hairpin loops, is essential for the hormone's biological activity. The loops are labelled αL1–3 on the α-chain, and βL1–3 on the β-chain. Other biologically important areas of the hormone are indicated. For clarity, the carbohydrate chains which are attached to the peptide have not been illustrated. The gonadotropins, LH and FSH, have a similar structure (from Szkudlinski M W, Fremont V, Ronin C et al. 2002. Thyroid-stimulating hormone and thyroid-stimulating hormone receptor structure–function relationships. Physiol Rev 82:473–502, with permission). (B) Growth hormone (i) and prolactin (ii). These are large, single-chain peptide hormones with disulphide bridges important in maintaining the tertiary structure of the hormones. Growth hormone and chorionic somatomammotropin (hCS) are very similar. The additional residues shown alongside the main chain show where hCS differs from growth hormone. (C) ACTH is a relatively small peptide hormone, consisting of just one chain of 39 amino acids. However, all of the biological activity is retained within the first 24 amino acids. ACTH is not glycosylated and there are no disulphide bridges.

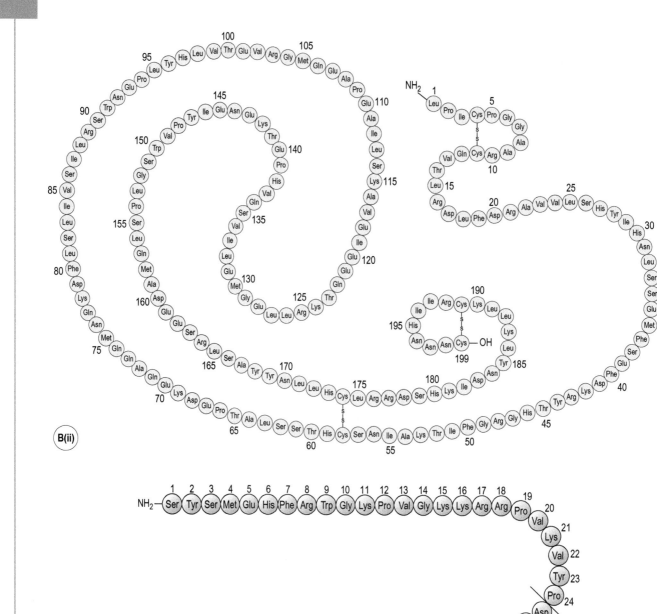

Figure 4.2 (Continued)

Interesting fact

Beta-endorphin (named as an abbreviation for 'endogenous morphine') is a 31 amino acid peptide which acts as an agonist at opioid receptors, principally μ1 and μ2. Beta-endorphin is produced as a neurotransmitter in the brain and spinal cord, where it has a role in mediating changes in neuronal excitability. It has been suggested that, as a neurotransmitter, it acts as a 'natural pain-reliever', with effects including analgesia and euphoria. However, what is even less clear is beta-endorphin's role as a hormone. It is released from the corticotroph cells of the anterior pituitary into the circulation but cannot cross the blood brain barrier to act on the brain because it is too large, although there is a possibility that an, as yet unidentified, mechanism exists for transporting beta-endorphin across the blood brain barrier. Beta endorphin does not have any clearly-identified action outside the brain although it has been suggested that it may have a role in regulating insulin release. There is still a lack of hard evidence to support the role of beta-endorphin, either as a neurotransmitter or a hormone, in the 'endorphin rush' experienced as a result of extreme physical effort, pain or danger.

Pro-opiomelanocortin

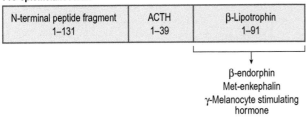

N-terminal peptide fragment 1–131	ACTH 1–39	β-Lipotrophin 1–91

β-endorphin
Met-enkephalin
γ-Melanocyte stimulating hormone

Figure 4.3 Pro-opiomelanocortin is a large precursor peptide that gives rise to a number of biologically active peptides, including β-endorphin, involved in the endogenous control of pain, and ACTH, the major regulator of adrenal function. The N-terminal fragment is thought to have a role in stimulating adrenal growth.

Regulation of hormone secretion in the anterior pituitary

The secretion of each of the anterior pituitary peptides is under a complex control system, involving both negative feedback and hypothalamic regulation by factors released from the hypothalamus into the portal system supplying the anterior pituitary. Most of the anterior pituitary hormones are regulated by 'stimulating factors' from the hypothalamus, but both growth hormone and prolactin are also regulated by hypothalamic 'release-inhibiting factors'. Most of the hypothalamic releasing and release-inhibiting factors are peptide hormones (Table 4.2 and Fig. 4.4), but some neurotransmitters, such as dopamine, are also involved.

Growth hormone and prolactin

The gene encoding growth hormone is located on the long arm of chromosome 17. In fact there is a family of genes encoding different forms of 'growth hormones' located in a

Case 4.1 Acromegaly: 2

Case history 2

The full history revealed that Mr Roberts had slowly and insidiously developed swelling of the hands and feet over about 5 years. He was no longer able to wear his wedding ring and had had to buy larger shoes. He complained of pins and needles in his hands and increased sweating, both particularly at night. In the last few years he had noted pain in the left hip on walking.

On examination, Mr Roberts had large hands and feet with thick doughy palms. His jaw was large and the lower teeth protruded in front of the upper teeth (Fig. 4.5). His tongue was large and his teeth were widely separated. His chest was large and shaped like a barrel and his blood pressure was 155/95 mmHg.

The blood tests showed a plasma glucose level of 12 mmol/L, but normal electrolytes, renal and liver function, and blood count.

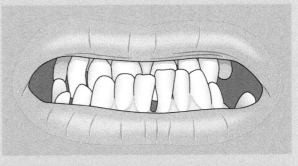

Figure 4.5 In acromegaly, the excess growth hormone causes the lower mandible, a flat bone, to grow. This causes the lower teeth to protrude beyond the upper teeth. Acromegaly may initially be noticed by the dentist, when a patient's teeth change or dentures no longer fit.

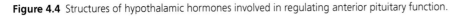

Hormone	Structure
Thyrotropin releasing hormone (TRH)	(pyro)Glu – His – Pro – NH₂
Gonadotropin releasing hormone (GnRH)	(pyro)Glu – His – Trp – Ser – Tyr – Gly – Leu – Arg – Pro – Gly – NH₂
Somatostatin	Ala – Gly – Cys – Lys – Asn– Phe – Phe – Trp – Lys – Thr – Phe – Thr – Ser – Cys (with S–S bridge between the two Cys)
Growth hormone releasing hormone (GHRH)	Tyr – Ala – Asp – Ala – Ile – Phe – Thr – Asn – Ser – Tyr – Arg – Lys – Val – Leu – Gly – Gln –Leu – Ser – Ala – Arg – Lys – Leu – Leu –Gln – Asp – Ile – Met – Ser – Arg – Gln – Gln – Gly – Glu – Ser – Asn – Gln – Glu – Arg – Gly – Ala – Arg – Ala –Arg – Leu – NH₂
Dopamine (inhibits prolactin secretion)	HO and HO on ring – CH₂CH₂NH₂
Corticotropin releasing hormone (CRH)	Ser – Gln – Glu – Pro – Pro – Ile – Ser – Leu – Asp – Leu – Thr – Phe – His – Leu – Leu – Arg – Glu – Val – Leu – Glu – Met – Thr – Lys –Ala – Asp – Gln – Leu – Ala – Gln – Gln – Ala – His – Ser – Asn – Arg – Lys – Leu – Leu – Asp – Ile – Ala – NH₂
Arginine vasopressin	Cys – Tyr – Phe – Gln – Asn – Cys – Pro – Arg – Gly – NH₂ (with S–S bridge between the two Cys)

Figure 4.4 Structures of hypothalamic hormones involved in regulating anterior pituitary function.

Table 4.2 Major hypothalamic factors and their actions

Hormone	Acronym	Structure[a]	Action
Thyrotropin releasing hormone	TRH	3	↑ TSH release
Gonadotropin releasing hormone	GnRH	10	↑ LH and FSH release
Corticotropin releasing hormone	CRH	41	↑ ACTH release
Arginine vasopressin	AVP	8	↑ ACTH release
Growth hormone releasing hormone	GHRH	44	↑ GH release
Somatostatin		14	↓ GH release
Dopamine		Catecholamine	↓ Prolactin release

[a]Number of amino acids.

cluster in this region. The main circulating form of growth hormone, however, is a 22 KDa single-chain polypeptide comprising 191 amino acids and with a tertiary structure maintained by two disulphide bridges (Fig. 4.2). A variant growth hormone gene is expressed in the placenta and encodes a peptide that differs from normal growth hormone in only 13 amino acids. In addition, this gene cluster encodes two variants of human placental lactogen (hPL1 and hPL2) also known as human chorionic somatomammotropin, a hormone related to growth hormone which is produced in pregnancy.

Prolactin is structurally very similar to growth hormone (Fig. 4.2) and shares a common evolutionary ancestor. It comprises 199 amino acids although only 16% are shared with growth hormone. Its tertiary structure is maintained with three disulphide bridges. Despite the ancestral relationship to growth hormone, the gene encoding prolactin is not found in the growth hormone gene cluster but is instead located on chromosome 6.

Regulation of growth hormone secretion

The hypothalamus secretes two peptides that exert opposing effects and together regulate growth hormone secretion (Fig. 4.6). Growth hormone releasing hormone (GHRH) stimulates growth hormone release, acting via specific G-protein linked GHRH receptors which increase intracellular cAMP, whereas somatostatin exerts an inhibitory effect by decreasing cAMP production. It is the balance between these two hormones that principally determines the rate of growth hormone secretion, although there is also direct metabolic regulation of GH secretion by blood levels of glucose and amino acids. In addition, there is interaction between other hormones and drugs and growth hormone secretion. In particular, dopamine and alpha-adrenergic agonists stimulate growth hormone release. Normal levels of growth hormone secretion require a normally- functioning thyroid gland and both under- and over-activity of the thyroid gland result in impaired growth hormone secretion. The gut peptide ghrelin also stimulates growth hormone secretion. It is thought that the effects of ghrelin to stimulate appetite, together with the ghrelin-induced rise in growth

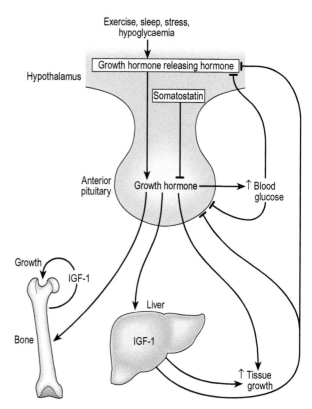

Figure 4.6 The regulation of growth hormone (GH) secretion. Two hypothalamic hormones regulate GH secretion: growth hormone releasing hormone and somatostatin. The balance between these hormones determines the rate of GH secretion. GH exerts many of its effects indirectly, through the production and action of IGF-1.

hormone, may act to coordinate the intake of nutrients with the stimulation of growth. Interestingly, growth hormone secretion is significantly reduced in obese individuals, although following weight loss normal levels of growth hormone secretion are restored.

There is also a negative feedback component in the regulation of growth hormone secretion, both by growth hormone itself and by insulin-like growth factor 1 (IGF-1) (see below). These feedback effects are on both the hypothalamus and the pituitary. There is also a short

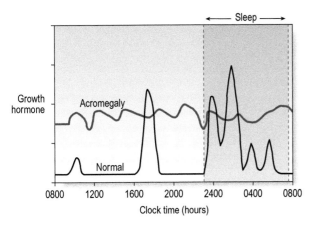

Figure 4.7 Diurnal pattern of GH secretion. During the day GH levels are often too low to measure. Secretion of GH increases during periods of sleep, particularly at the start of sleep, and there are also 'spikes' of secretion during the day. The secretion of GH is described as 'episodic'. In acromegaly, there is less variation in GH levels throughout the day and the level of GH never becomes undetectable. The plasma half-life of GH is about 30 min.

feedback loop in the hypothalamus whereby GHRH inhibits its own secretion.

A major physiological stimulus for growth hormone secretion is the onset of sleep. In both adults and children there is a marked diurnal variation in growth hormone secretion with a peak occurring 1–2h after the onset of sleep (Fig. 4.7). The effect of sleep on growth hormone secretion is greatest in children and declines with increasing age. The secretion of growth hormone is also stimulated by stress, exercise, the presence of certain amino acids in plasma (especially arginine) and by a fall in plasma glucose concentrations. It is suppressed by high plasma glucose levels. These effects can be used clinically to investigate disorders of growth hormone secretion. Such dynamic testing for growth hormone is significant because the secretion of growth hormone is episodic and so a single-point measurement is of limited clinical value.

Regulation of prolactin secretion

Prolactin is unique among the major hormones in that its secretion is mainly under inhibitory control. Experimentally, several hormones have been shown to stimulate prolactin release, and for a long time there was a search for 'the prolactin releasing factor'. It is now clear, however, that prolactin secretion is under tonic inhibitory control, principally by dopamine released from the hypothalamus. If the inhibitory effect of dopamine is removed then secretion of prolactin occurs (Fig. 4.9). Of less physiological significance, there are also several factors which stimulate prolactin release, the most potent of which is thyrotropin releasing hormone, TRH. There is a short negative feedback loop involving prolactin itself causing an increase in hypothalamic dopamine levels.

The major physiological stimulus to prolactin secretion is suckling. Prolactin levels also rise during the latter

Case 4.1 Acromegaly: 3

Case note: Establishing the diagnosis
Measurement of serum growth hormone

Normally growth hormone secretion is controlled by a negative feedback loop involving IGF-1. However, in acromegaly the pituitary adenoma secretes growth hormone in a manner that is relatively resistant to feedback regulation. In addition to higher levels of growth hormone, the pattern of secretion is altered. Normally, growth hormone is secreted at night and is often undetectable during the day, whereas in acromegaly pulses of growth hormone are made throughout the night and day, the diurnal rhythm is lost, and growth hormone is never undetectable (Fig. 4.7). To confirm the diagnosis, growth hormone will be found in detectable amounts during the day and serum IGF-1 levels will be high.

Oral glucose test (Fig. 4.8)

This is very similar to the test used to confirm diabetes mellitus. A fixed dose of glucose is given orally after an overnight fast and serum hormone levels are measured at intervals. Oral glucose normally suppresses growth hormone to undetectable levels, but in acromegaly the levels are not suppressible.

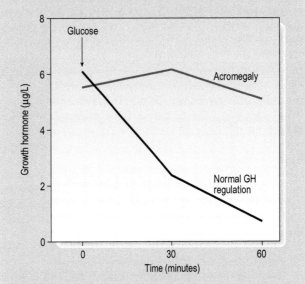

Figure 4.8 Glucose suppression of GH secretion. An oral dose of glucose is given after a period of fasting. Blood GH levels are measured at 0, 30 and 60 min after the glucose load. In a normal person, the level of GH should be lower than 2 μg/L at 30 and 60 min. In a person with acromegaly the GH is not suppressed and may even show a paradoxical increase.

half of pregnancy, an effect that is thought to be mediated by oestradiol. Like growth hormone, prolactin secretion is also increased during sleep and by stress and exercise. However prolactin secretion is not linked to a particular phase of the sleep cycle.

4

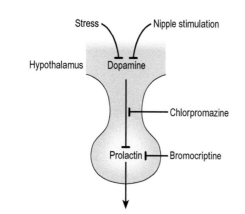

Figure 4.9 Regulation of prolactin secretion. Prolactin is under *tonic inhibitory control* by dopamine. This means that prolactin is released only when dopamine secretion by the hypothalamus is inhibited. Drugs that mimic dopamine, such as bromocriptine, inhibit prolactin, but dopamine *antagonists*, such as chlorpromazine, stimulate prolactin release. There does not appear to be any negative feedback regulation in the control of prolactin secretion.

Growth hormone and prolactin in blood

Growth hormone is unusual among peptide hormones because it has a plasma binding protein. About 50% of the circulating growth hormone is bound to growth hormone binding protein (GHBP). This protein is not like the other hormone binding proteins, which are globins secreted by the liver. The GHBP is a protein cleaved from the extracellular domain of the growth hormone receptor, so is released from growth hormone target tissues. It is known that GHBP levels vary with changes in hormonal status. It appears to function in the same way as other hormone binding proteins, protecting the hormone from metabolic degradation, reducing the renal clearance of growth hormone and providing a readily accessible plasma pool of hormone. It has been suggested that GHBP may compete with growth hormone receptors, but the significance of this is not clear. Interestingly, in patients with growth hormone insensitivity (Laron syndrome), GHBP measurement may be used as a diagnostic tool. GHBP is low or undetectable in around three quarters of patients with Laron syndrome.

It has been suggested that a prolactin binding protein may also circulate but this remains speculative.

The plasma half-life of both prolactin and growth hormone is around 20–40 min.

Actions of the anterior pituitary hormones growth: hormone and prolactin

Actions of growth hormone

Growth hormone exerts some direct hormonal effects, but many of its actions are indirect, mediated by another hormone (Fig. 4.6) called insulin-like growth factor 1 (IGF-1, pronounced I-G-F-one). It can be argued that the main action of growth hormone is in stimulating the production

Box 4.1 Stress hormones

Several of the anterior pituitary hormones are known as 'stress hormones' as their secretion increases in response to stress. These include ACTH, growth hormone, prolactin and to some extent TSH. The 'stress' can be either physical, such as exercise, or psychological, such as exam stress. Paradigms exist for testing different forms of stress under laboratory conditions; the standard psychological stressor is performing mental arithmetic in front of an audience. Standard physiological stressors include the cold stressor test which involves plunging your arm into a bucket of ice water for a fixed period of time. Other stressors that stimulate the secretion of these hormones include exercise, hypoglycaemia induced by insulin administration (see below), sleep deprivation, infection and pyrexia. Non-pituitary stress hormones include the adrenal hormones: glucocorticoids and adrenaline and noradrenaline.

of this growth factor, IGF-1, by the liver. Together, growth hormone and IGF-1 regulate tissue growth and several metabolic pathways.

Growth hormone receptors

The effects of growth hormone are mediated by the growth hormone receptor, which is a member of the recently characterized family of cytokine receptors (see Ch. 2). Mutations of the gene encoding the growth hormone receptor result in low IGF-1 levels and significantly reduced growth (Laron syndrome). Growth hormone receptors are located in tissues throughout the body, but most significantly in liver, muscle and adipose tissue. In all tissues, the growth hormone receptor signals through the JAK-STAT pathway (see Ch. 2 for details).

Insulin-like growth factor-1

IGF-1 is a member of a family of growth factors which are structurally closely related to pro-insulin. Indeed the similarity is so great that IGF-1 can bind to and activate insulin receptors. The peptide family has two members, IGF-1, the adult form, and IGF-2, the major fetal form.

One of the key actions of growth hormone is to stimulate the production of IGF-1, an action which requires the presence of insulin. In general, IGF-1 concentrations correlate well with growth hormone concentrations, except when there is a receptor defect, such as in Laron syndrome, when growth hormone levels are relatively high and IGF-1 low. Many tissues produce IGF-1 in response to growth hormone stimulation, and IGF-1 has both autocrine and paracrine actions in many tissues. In bone, growth hormone, parathyroid hormone and oestrogens all stimulate IGF-1 release. The liver is the major source of IGF-1 in the circulation. In blood, IGF-1 circulates bound to an IGF binding protein (IGFBP). This binding protein is thought to account for the relatively long plasma half-life of IGF, which is around 12h. A third protein, called acid labile subunit, also binds to IGF and its binding protein in plasma. Together this complex transports IGF around the body, possibly accounting for the ability of IGF-1 to cross the blood brain barrier, and also regulates the bioavailability of IGF-1. Various tissues, and particularly some tumour tissues, produce a protease which acts on IGFBP and so causes a local increase in the concentration of free IGF-1. As IGF-1 stimulates cell division, this has clear implications for tumour growth.

Effects of growth hormone and IGF-1

Growth

Both growth hormone and IGF-1 circulate to the tissues to cause growth of nearly every organ and tissue. In prepubertal children, before fusion of the epiphyses, growth hormone, via the actions of IGF-1, stimulates long bone growth and is the major hormone responsible for linear growth, although thyroxine is also required for growth to take place (Fig. 4.10). In the absence of growth hormone there is a failure of linear growth (see below). IGF-1 has several actions which increase the growth of bone: it regulates the activity of chondrocytes, the cells responsible for laying down cartilage; it stimulates osteoblast cell division; and it increases the synthesis of both collagen and bone matrix. Overall IGF-1 has a major effect on stimulating bone growth.

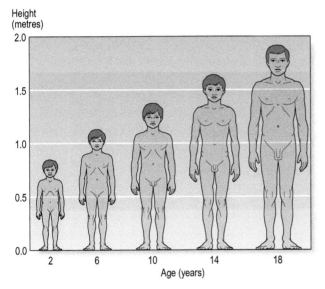

Figure 4.10 Growth hormone is responsible for the normal increase in height through childhood. In the absence of GH, linear growth is severely limited. A typical height for a 10-year-old boy with a severe GH deficiency would be about 1 m. However, most cases would be diagnosed at a much earlier age than this.

Metabolism

Growth hormone also has a range of metabolic effects, acting to raise blood glucose and free fatty acid concentrations, while promoting protein synthesis in muscle (Table 4.3). Metabolic effects of growth hormone include:

- *Protein metabolism*: increases amino acid uptake and protein synthesis in muscle

- *Carbohydrate metabolism*: stimulates gluconeogenesis, decreases peripheral glucose utilization. Generally antagonizes insulin actions

- *Lipid metabolism*: stimulates release of free fatty acids and glycerol from adipose tissue.

Table 4.3 Metabolic effects of growth hormone and IGF-1

Metabolic measure	GH	IGF-1
Plasma glucose levels	↑	↓
Hepatic gluconeogenesis	↑	↓
Hepatic glycogenesis	↑	↓
Insulin sensitivity	↓	↑
Glucose uptake (muscle, etc.)	↓	↑
Lipolysis	↑	↓
Protein synthesis (muscle, etc.)	↑	↑

The effects of IGF-1 are very similar to those of insulin as they are each able to bind to both receptors. In general, the effects of GH oppose those of insulin. However, both IGF-1 and GH act to increase protein synthesis in muscle.

Interesting fact

Some endurance athletes, such as swimmers and cyclists, try to exploit the action of growth hormone on muscle by using it as a performance-enhancing drug. They take injections of recombinant growth hormone in order to increase their muscle bulk and in the hope that it will be less easily detected than anabolic steroids.

Actions of prolactin

Receptors for prolactin are located in many tissues including breast, liver, ovary and prostate. Prolactin receptors bind growth hormone with nearly equal affinity. Prolactin is the major hormone of lactation, acting on the oestrogen-primed breast to initiate and maintain lactation. Glucocorticoids have a permissive role in lactation, as does the decrease in oestrogen and progesterone levels postpartum.

Prolactin and growth hormone have a role in the very complex control of breast development in adolescent girls. Oestrogen, progesterone and adrenal steroids are also required, together with insulin and thyroid hormones. Breast development in males is inhibited by testosterone.

In addition, prolactin inhibits ovulation, by inhibiting gonadotropin releasing hormone (GnRH) secretion from the hypothalamus and it is quite normal for a woman who is breastfeeding to have no menstrual cycle until either the child is weaned or the frequency of feeding is insufficient to maintain prolactin levels at high enough concentrations to maintain this inhibitory effect. This effect of prolactin explains why breastfeeding has long been used as natural contraception by many women.

The prolactin receptor, like the growth hormone receptor is a member of the cytokine receptor superfamily, which signals through the JAK-STAT pathway (see Ch. 2). There are receptors for prolactin in the liver, ovary and prostate, but their physiological significance is not known. The physiological function of prolactin in men is also unclear.

> **Interesting fact**
>
> In the USA, growth hormone is widely used in dairy farming. It strongly stimulates lactation and is used to increase the volume of milk yielded by each cow. It is also used to 'bulk-up' beef cattle more rapidly. The proponents of this type of farming are keen to point out that there is no danger to human health from this practice. The European Union, however, has banned all growth hormone products in both dairy and beef farming.

Disorders of anterior pituitary function: over-secretion

Pituitary adenomas, tumours of the anterior pituitary that secrete hormones, are relatively uncommon. However, when they do occur they have profound effects on the body. A corticotroph adenoma, secreting ACTH, causes adrenal hyperfunction, resulting in 'Cushing's disease'. A thyrotroph adenoma causes hyperthyroidism, whereas a gonadotroph adenoma affects ovarian and testicular function. These will be considered in more detail in the chapters covering those endocrine systems. In this chapter, we will focus on growth hormone and prolactin.

Excess growth hormone secretion

This is most often caused by a secretory tumour (adenoma) of the pituitary somatotroph cells. As with other conditions of excess hormone secretion, the effects seen are an exaggeration of the normal physiological effects of the hormone. In children, the effect of excess growth hormone is an increase in linear growth, particularly of the long bones, resulting in a condition of extreme height, termed giantism. In adults, excess growth hormone secretion causes acromegaly, a condition easily recognized in its later stages by the characteristic growth of the hands, feet and lower jaw (Fig. 4.11). The effects on the lower jaw can cause gaps between teeth, a diagnostic feature which is often spotted by dentists. There is often a coarsening of the facial features, with increased growth of the lips and nose and of the skin above the eyes. The onset of symptoms is usually slow and there is often a delay of several years between the onset of acromegaly and first presentation at an endocrine clinic. The other effects of acromegaly are rather more serious than the visible cosmetic changes: there is growth of the viscera which particularly affects the heart and cardiovascular system. There are also metabolic changes which include impaired glucose tolerance, caused by the general anti-insulin effects of growth hormone to decrease

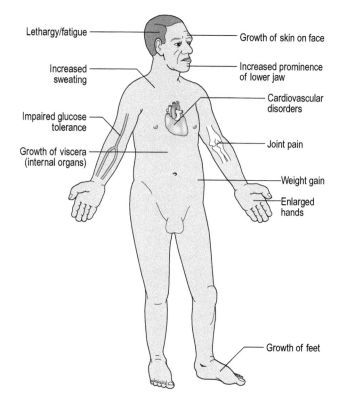

Figure 4.11 Signs and symptoms of acromegaly (excessive growth hormone secretion in an adult).

> ### Case 4.1   Acromegaly: 4
>
> #### Case note: Explanation of symptoms
>
> The actions of growth hormone and IGF-1 affect all organs and soft tissues (Fig. 4.11). Long bones are also capable of growth if the growth plates are unfused. This occurs when the tumour develops before puberty, and results in tall stature, or giantism. The effect of excess growth hormone and IGF-1 on the joints is to accelerate arthritis by over-stimulation of cartilage and peri-articular bone. The internal organs also grow and cardiac hypertrophy and high blood pressure result. Sweating is due to growth of the skin and the sweat glands. Growth of the soft tissue surrounding the median nerve results in compression under the carpal tunnel, with bilateral carpal tunnel syndrome causing painful tingling and weakness of the hands, especially at night.
>
> Growth hormone is also one of the three major hormones that counter the action of insulin; the other two are cortisol and glucagon. Thus, impaired glucose tolerance and diabetes are common in acromegaly. This explains Mr Roberts' high glucose concentration.
>
> Growth of the lower jaw and tongue made anaesthesia difficult and the teeth may be loose. Mr Roberts' acromegaly should be controlled or treated before other non-urgent surgery (such as his hernia repair) takes place.

peripheral glucose utilization and increase hepatic gluconeogenesis. This diabetogenic effect of excess growth hormone contributes to the increased cardiovascular risk. As a result, premature death from cardiovascular disorders is a significant risk in acromegaly.

Treatment of acromegaly

The first-line treatment of acromegaly is surgical removal of the tumour by transsphenoidal surgery. Radiotherapy may also be used to either remove or shrink the tumour. A somatostatin analogue, called octreotide, is also used to treat acromegaly. It can be used to shrink a tumour prior to surgery, or to control symptoms while waiting for radiotherapy to become effective. Octreotide can also be used when the first-line treatment has failed to bring about a decrease in plasma IGF-1 levels. It is a long-acting preparation, so even though it has to be injected, it is effective for 4 weeks. Somatostatin has a wide range of effects in the body, especially in the gastrointestinal system and adverse effects of octreotide therapy can include gastrointestinal disturbances.

A new area for therapeutic intervention in acromegaly is the development of growth hormone receptor (GHR) antagonists. The first of these to be licensed was pegvisomant, a PEGylated (see below) growth hormone analogue which acts as a GHR antagonist. It is only used when both first-line treatments of surgery or radiotherapy have not been effective and second-line treatment with somatostatin analogues fails to reduce IGF-1 levels to normal, or is not tolerated. Because pegvisomant is a modified peptide, it has to be given by subcutaneous injection, usually once daily.

Interesting fact

PEGylation is the covalent binding of PEG (pronounced 'peg') to a target molecule such as a protein. PEG is poly(ethylene glycol), a non-toxic and non-immunogenic polymer which is readily metabolized in the body (and not to be confused with ethylene glycol, a toxic chemical used in antifreeze). PEGylation is particularly useful for peptides and proteins used therapeutically as it makes the molecule bigger and with altered physical and chemical properties. For example, PEGylated peptides are less antigenic as the long-chain polymers effectively cloak the peptide from the host immune system. They are also protected from proteolytic enzymes and their large size reduces renal clearance so their half-life in the circulation is prolonged. Other advantages include increased water solubility, greater stability in solution and the ability to engineer altered receptor affinity via induced conformational changes. As if all this was not enough, there is a further incentive for the pharmaceutical companies: PEGylation of a drug which is already licensed counts as a new drug product for patent purposes.

Excess prolactin secretion

Prolactinoma, a prolactin secreting tumour, is the most commonly occurring pituitary tumour. The presence of

---

Case 4.2   Hyperprolactinaemia: 1

Case history

The class of drugs most likely to cause hyperprolactinaemia is the neuroleptics, dopamine antagonists used to treat psychosis. Mr Green, a 46-year-old man with a long history of psychotic illness, had recently had his neuroleptic medication increased by his GP. At his next outpatient appointment with his psychiatrist, Mr Green appeared to have developed a new symptom. He had always had a variety of false beliefs that various government agencies were plotting against him, but had now become convinced that his GP was trying to turn him into a woman. When asked the standard question 'What evidence do you have for this?', he unbuttoned his shirt to reveal significant gynaecomastia and expressed milk from both breasts. His serum prolactin was 4,265 mU/L (normal range <400 mU/L). Three months after changing his neuroleptic medication his serum prolactin was normal, his gynaecomastia had resolved and he was back on speaking terms with his GP.

such a tumour causes hyperprolactinaemia, the condition of excess circulating prolactin concentrations. However, this condition may also result from other causes, particularly as an adverse effect of drugs that reduce dopaminergic transmission, especially antipsychotic drugs such as risperidone. In women, excess prolactin causes cessation of the menstrual cycle and may cause inappropriate lactation, termed galactorrhoea. In men, prolactin may also cause growth of breast tissue, termed gynaecomastia.

One unusual, but endocrinologically interesting, cause of hyperprolactinaemia is any space-occupying lesion, such as a tumour, in the pituitary fossa. Compression of the pituitary stalk cuts off the delivery of dopamine to the lactotrophs and, because dopamine inhibits prolactin secretion, the effect is to greatly increase prolactin secretion. This is called 'stalk disconnection syndrome'.

Where excess prolactin secretion is due to an adverse drug effect, it is usually possible to find an alternative medication which does not have this effect. For both idiopathic hyperprolactinaemia and prolactinomas, the first-line treatment is to use a dopamine agonist, such as cabergoline, to inhibit prolactin secretion and return blood levels to normal.

Disorders of under-secretion of anterior pituitary hormones

Hypopituitarism or under-secretion of pituitary hormones may occur as a result of trauma, infarction or surgical removal of the pituitary gland (hypophysectomy). As the pituitary gland occupies a space confined by bone, the presence of any tumour in the region is likely to cause compression and loss of pituitary function. Although most of the tumours of anterior pituitary cells cause symptoms by over-secretion of a particular hormone, these tumours are also likely to cause a loss of function of other cell types as the tumour compresses the cells. It is also possible to find non-functional tumours that are space occupying and cause an overall loss of anterior pituitary function termed panhypopituitarism.

There is a pattern to the effects of such space-occupying tumours on anterior pituitary function. Growth hormone is usually the first hormone to be lost, with LH/FSH next, and ACTH and TSH being the most resistant to damage. As noted above, there may be a paradoxical effect on prolactin secretion: if the pituitary stalk is compressed, then dopamine inhibition of lactotrophs is lost and prolactin secretion rises.

Panhypopituitarism is a serious condition, resulting in hypotension, hypoglycaemia, lethargy and weakness (Fig. 4.12). The loss of adrenal function due to lack of ACTH can be life threatening (see Ch. 6). There is also a loss of libido and secondary sex characteristics. In children, there is growth failure and failure to enter puberty.

Loss of anterior pituitary function means that replacement of some hormones is necessary. In particular, loss of ACTH and TSH results in loss of adrenal and thyroid function. As a general rule, it is not the pituitary hormones that are replaced, as these are all large peptides and would require frequent injection. Instead the thyroid hormone, thyroxine, and adrenal steroids are given as these both correct the deficiencies and are active orally.

In the case of the gonadotropins, LH and FSH, secondary sexual characteristics can be induced and maintained by oral administration of sex steroids. However, when a woman with hypopituitarism wishes to conceive, gonadotropins can be used to induce ovulation.

Interesting fact

A very rare, and therefore utterly memorable, cause of hypopituitarism is Sheehan's syndrome. This is caused by a sudden decrease in blood volume or a localized bleed disrupting the hypophyseal portal system. In the 'bad old days', Sheehan's syndrome was most often associated with blood loss in childbirth. Because the posterior pituitary has a separate arterial supply, Sheehan's syndrome affects only the anterior pituitary, resulting in loss of its hormone secretion.

Tests for hypopituitarism

The first investigation for hypofunction of the pituitary is to measure blood concentrations of the pituitary hormones at 0900 hours. However, more complex tests are sometimes needed. An insulin tolerance test can be used to check ACTH and growth hormone secretion; a tightly controlled dose of insulin is given to induce hypoglycaemia and the pituitary response is measured by checking levels of ACTH and GH. These hormones are both strongly stimulated by hypoglycaemia. Clearly, this is a potentially dangerous test and cannot be used in some patients, such as those with heart disease.

Insufficient growth hormone secretion

The effects of hyposecretion of growth hormone are most significant in children as growth hormone is necessary

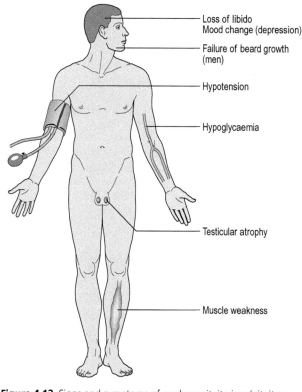

Loss of libido
Mood change (depression)

Failure of beard growth (men)

Hypotension

Hypoglycaemia

Testicular atrophy

Muscle weakness

Figure 4.12 Signs and symptoms of panhypopituitarism (pituitary insufficiency) in an adult.

Case 4.1 Acromegaly: 5

Case note: Further tests

The anterior pituitary controls other hormonal systems and these may be damaged by pressure or invasion by an anterior pituitary adenoma. An important axis for maintaining blood pressure is the pituitary–adrenal axis. This should be shown to be functioning normally (see Ch. 6) or, if not, be replaced by exogenous glucocorticoids before any surgical treatment of the acromegaly. The serum thyroxine and testosterone levels should also be measured to test the integrity of the pituitary–thyroid and pituitary–gonadal axes, respectively.

Occasionally, the prolactin level will be high. This may be because the adenoma secretes both prolactin and growth hormone. However, some tumours block the delivery of dopamine to the normal lactotroph, releasing it from tonic inhibition.

Case 4.1 Acromegaly: 6

Case note: Management

The main treatment of acromegaly is surgical removal of the adenoma. However, although 80% of small tumours (<1 cm in diameter) are curable by surgery, only 40% of tumours >1 cm are resectable. This means that additional treatments are needed. Radiotherapy is successful in reducing the size of the adenoma and the levels of growth hormone. However, radiotherapy may take several years for full effect. Medical treatments that may be needed include dopamine agonists and somatostatin analogues. The dopamine agonists work because the somatotroph and lactotroph share a similar cellular lineage and somatotroph adenomas may express dopamine receptors on the cell surface. Somatostatin is a hypothalamic peptide that lowers growth hormone secretion in physiological states. Synthetic analogues of somatostatin (e.g. octreotide, which contains eight somatostatin molecules) bind to adenomas and reduce their size and growth hormone secretion in a majority of cases.

The anatomy and relations of the pituitary are vital to the surgical cure of acromegaly. The surgeon approaches the pituitary fossa through the nose and the sphenoidal sinus. The operation must be performed by an experienced surgeon and a particular danger is entry into the cavernous sinuses which are blood-filled venous channels (rather like a sponge) lateral to the fossa. Severe bleeding may result from this error. Radiation therapy may be given, but is planned so that the dose of radiation given to the normal brain structures, in particular the optic chiasm, is as low as possible.

for normal growth during childhood. However, there are many reasons for failure of growth in children and growth hormone insufficiency is relatively uncommon. In adults, there is increasing evidence that growth hormone is necessary both for the maintenance of a normal body composition and to maintain wellbeing. In the absence of growth hormone there is an increase in body fat and a loss of muscle strength. Growth hormone deficiency is treated by daily injections of recombinant growth hormone. Growth hormone, like other pituitary peptides used therapeutically, used to be extracted from human or animal pituitary glands, but the possible transmission of prion diseases made this undesirable. At the same time, modern molecular technology has made it possible to produce relatively large amounts of this and other hormones safely.

Interesting fact

If you type 'HGH releaser' into an internet search engine, you will find many websites advertising products that are claimed not only to raise your growth hormone levels, but also to stop you from ageing, increase your lean body mass, improve your sex drive and generally bring peace on earth. Using your new-found knowledge of the endocrinology of the pituitary and growth hormone, ask yourself to what extent these claims can be justified. For example, would growth hormone be active if taken orally? Would amino acid mixtures designed to stimulate the pituitary be likely to raise growth hormone above physiological levels? How much money can you make selling these products?

THE ADRENAL GLANDS PART I: THE ADRENAL MEDULLA

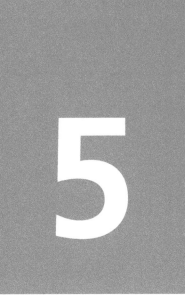

Chapter objectives

After studying this chapter you should be able to:

1. Describe the structure of the adrenal glands and understand how the inner (medulla) and outer (cortex) parts of each gland have separate functions.

2. Describe the development of the adrenal glands.

3. Describe the function of the adrenal medulla including the synthesis, secretion and actions of the medullary hormones.

4. Explain what is meant by a phaeochromocytoma and describe how it is diagnosed and treated.

Introduction

Each adrenal gland is really two quite separate glands. The much larger outer part is the adrenal cortex, which produces steroid hormones (cortisol, aldosterone and androgens), and the smaller inner part is the adrenal medulla, which produces catecholamines (principally adrenaline). Although they have different functions, the cortex and medulla share a common blood supply and both have an important role in the body's response to stress. The hormones of the adrenal medulla are involved in the very short-term 'fight or flight' response, while the cortical hormones have a longer-term homeostatic role, which enables the body to cope with stress.

Where to find the adrenal glands

There are two adrenal glands, each situated on the superior pole of the kidney, embedded in the perirenal fat (Fig. 5.1). They are roughly triangular in shape and each weighs about 4 g in the adult. The adrenal cortical tissue totally surrounds the inner medulla, and is arranged in three concentric zones, called the zona glomerulosa, zona fasciculata and zona reticularis (Fig. 5.2).

Interesting fact

Although there are two adrenal glands, if one is damaged or removed the other rapidly increases in size and takes over the function of the damaged gland. So you can lose the function of one adrenal gland without any adverse effects, but losing both adrenal glands may be rapidly fatal unless cortisol is given regularly.

Blood supply

The adrenal gland is a highly vascular organ: virtually every cell is in direct contact with a blood vessel. The adrenal glands receive blood from the adrenal arteries,

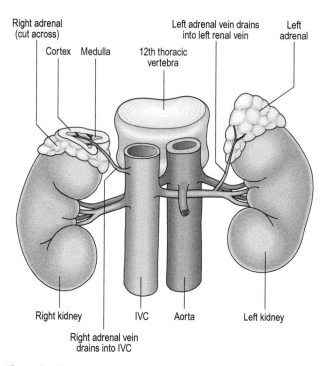

Figure 5.1 Diagram to show the anatomical relations of the adrenal glands and their blood supply. The arterial supply to the adrenals is via small arterioles that arise directly from the aorta. Note that the right adrenal vein drains directly into the inferior vena cava (IVC), whereas the left adrenal vein drains into the left renal vein.

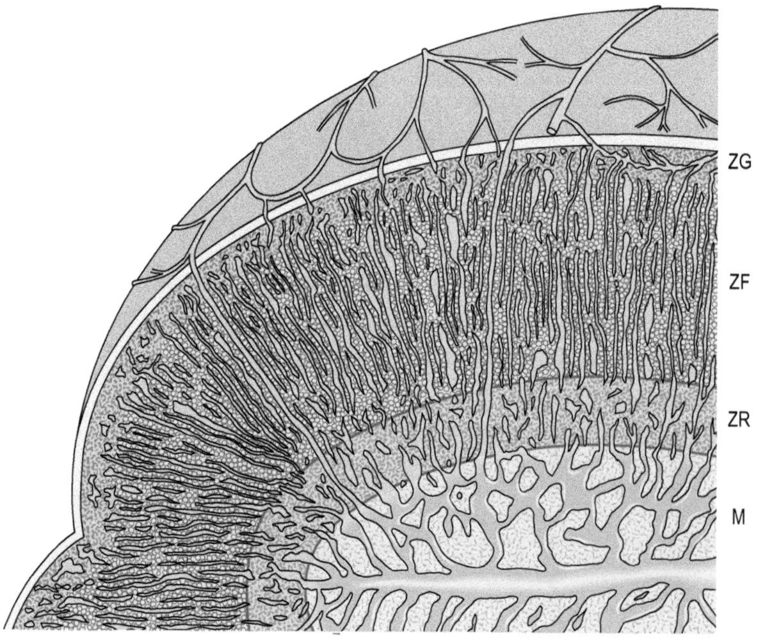

Figure 5.2 Cross-section through the adrenal gland to show the relationship between the adrenal cortex and the medulla. ZG, zona glomerulosa; ZF, zona fasciculata; ZR, zona reticularis. Together, these three zones comprise the adrenal cortex. M, adrenal medulla.

which arise directly from the aorta (Fig. 5.1). After they pass through the connective tissue capsule of the adrenal, these arteries form an arteriolar network (arteriolar plexus). This gives rise to a small number of medullary arteries which pass directly through the cortex to the medulla, and a very large number of tiny thin-walled blood vessels, called sinusoids, which pass through the layers of the adrenal cortex into the medulla. Here, the sinusoids merge, eventually forming a single large central vein, the adrenal vein, which exits through the cortex. This drains into the left renal vein from the left adrenal gland, but directly into the vena cava from the right.

The importance of the adrenal glands to the body's normal functioning is shown by the fact that, in states of circulatory collapse, the blood supply to the adrenals is preserved. In fact, only the blood supply to the brain is as well protected from interruption. The adrenal medulla receives most of its blood supply through the cortical sinusoids and only a very small proportion through the medullary arteries. Because the cells of the adrenal cortex are arranged alongside sinusoids, into which they secrete their steroid products, the cells of the medulla are constantly bathed in steroid-rich blood.

Interesting fact

The drainage of the short right adrenal vein directly into the inferior vena cava can make it difficult for a surgeon to perform a right adrenalectomy safely. On the other hand, there is a risk of damaging the spleen during a left adrenalectomy. If you are having both adrenals removed, choose your surgeon carefully!

Nerve supply

The adrenal medulla is a modified ganglion of the sympathetic nervous system. Instead of noradrenaline being released into the synaptic cleft as a neurotransmitter, it is released into the circulation as a hormone. The adrenal innervation is via the splanchnic nerves, which come from the spinal cord at levels D8–D11. Conventionally, it is said that the splanchnic nerve passes directly through the cortex to innervate the adrenal medulla but in fact there is also a significant nerve supply to the cortex.

Embryology of the adrenal gland

As you might expect from their completely different structure and function, the two parts of the adrenal develop from different tissues. The cells of the adrenal cortex are mesodermal in origin, whereas those of the medulla are derived from the neural crest and migrate into the cortical tissue during fetal development. The fetal adrenal is relatively large, reaching the size of the adult gland at birth. Most of the bulk of the fetal adrenal comprises a special zone, called the fetal zone. The role of the fetal zone appears to be mainly the production of precursor steroids that can

Case 5.1 Phaeochromocytoma: 1

Case history

Mrs Smith was a 45-year-old woman who was urgently referred by her GP to the duty medical team at the local hospital, with a 2-week history of sweating and palpitations. She described sudden episodes of rapid heart beating, lasting for 10–15 min and occurring at least once an hour. She had been worried that these might be panic attacks as she felt very frightened during these episodes. The GP thought the same until he checked her pulse rate and blood pressure.

On examination, Mrs Smith was pale, with a pulse rate of 100/min, and blood pressure fluctuating between 155/105 and 260/165 mmHg. Investigations gave the following results:

Serum sodium	141 mmol/L (normal, 136–146 mmol/L)
Serum potassium	3.2 mmol/L (normal, 3.5–4.5 mmol/L)
Plasma noradrenaline	12 nmol/L (normal, <5 nmol/L)
Plasma adrenaline	6.7 nmol/L (normal, <1.5 nmol/L).

be metabolized to oestriol, an oestrogen, by the placenta. This zone disappears rapidly after birth and the adrenal gland decreases in size. The adrenal glands then increase in size during childhood, in proportion to the rest of the body.

The adrenal medulla

Introduction

The adrenal medulla is at the interface between the neural and endocrine systems and has features of both. The hormones of the adrenal medulla are the catecholamines, which also function as classical neurotransmitters in the autonomic nervous system. The adrenal medulla itself is modified neural tissue and its activity is regulated by a direct neural input. So the medulla functions like a modified sympathetic ganglion. However, the catecholamines of the adrenal medulla are released into blood, rather than a synaptic cleft, and act at sites distant from the site of secretion, by activating specific receptors. So the adrenal medulla also functions like a conventional endocrine gland. However, the actions of the medullary hormones are far more rapid and short-lived than those of most hormones. In these ways the adrenal medulla and its hormones really do lie at the interface between hormonal and neural communication.

Structure

The adrenal medulla is the innermost part of the adrenal gland and comprises modified neural tissue. The cells of the adrenal medulla are called 'chromaffin' cells. This term was coined by a Czech biologist, Alfred Kohn, early in the 20th century because of their affinity for chromium compounds. Histological stains containing chromium salts form a characteristic brownish colour in the cells. Structurally the cells of the adrenal medulla are easily distinguished from those of the cortex: they have no lipid droplets but instead contain numerous secretory granules. The gross appearance of the adrenal medulla is considerably darker than the surrounding cortex.

Interesting fact

The cells of the adrenal medulla degrade very rapidly after death and form a dark coloured liquid centre to the adrenal glands. Because of this, in 1611 the Danish anatomist Bairtholinus was able to confidently describe the function of the adrenals as being the production of black bile. It was only in the 19th century that the French scientist George Cuvier 'discovered' the cells of the adrenal medulla.

The hormones of the adrenal medulla

The chromaffin cells of the adrenal medulla secrete catecholamines, adrenaline (also called epinephrine), noradrenaline (also called norepinephrine) and dopamine, which are synthesized from the amino acid tyrosine (Fig. 5.3). The major product of the human adrenal medulla is adrenaline, whereas noradrenaline is more abundant in the central and sympathetic nervous systems. The processes of catecholamine synthesis and release are the same in the adrenal medulla as in the rest of the nervous system. The rate limiting step of catecholamine synthesis is the conversion of tyrosine to dihydroxyphenylalanine, catalysed by the enzyme tyrosine hydroxylase. The enzyme which converts noradrenaline to adrenaline, phenylethanolamine-N-methyltransferase (PNMT), is regulated by glucocorticoids, so the fact that the medullary cells are bathed in steroid-rich blood maintains the expression of this enzyme and the high proportion of adrenaline secreted. If steroid secretion by the adrenal cortex is blocked, then the medulla shrinks in size and secretes mostly noradrenaline. The catecholamines, once synthesized, are stored in granules in preparation for release.

In addition to the catecholamines, the adrenal medulla secretes a range of peptide hormones, including the opiate peptides met-enkephalin and leu-enkephalin. It also secretes adrenomedullin, a peptide involved in blood pressure regulation (see Ch. 13), arginine vasopressin and vasoactive intestinal peptide. Some of these peptides have been shown to have stimulatory effects on catecholamine secretion when tested in the laboratory. However, their physiological function in the adrenal medulla remains unclear.

Regulation of catecholamine secretion

The activity of the adrenal medulla is regulated by the activity of the splanchnic nerve. The neurotransmitter in

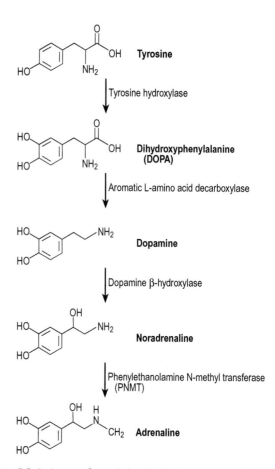

Figure 5.3 Pathways of catecholamine biosynthesis in the adrenal medulla. The final enzyme in the pathway, PNMT, is regulated by glucocorticoids.

the adrenal medulla is acetylcholine which acts on nicotinic receptors. Acetylcholine release is increased in response to pain, anxiety and trauma as well as exercise and hypoglycaemia. Acetylcholine acts to increase the rate of catecholamine synthesis and also stimulates the release of catecholamine-containing storage granules. Basal circulating levels of adrenaline are around 0.1 to 0.5 nmol/L and of noradrenaline are around 1 to 2.5 nmol/L in healthy people at rest. These levels can increase 10-fold following exercise. The major secretory product of the human adrenal medulla is adrenaline. The reason that circulating noradrenaline levels are so much higher than adrenaline is because most of the noradrenaline in blood comes from other post-ganglionic nerve terminals.

Transport and metabolism of adrenal medullary hormones

In contrast to most hormones, the effects of catecholamines are very rapid and short-lived, with a half-life in plasma of seconds. There is no specific plasma binding protein for these hormones but instead the catecholamines circulate bound to plasma albumin.

Table 5.1 Effects of adrenoceptor activation

Receptor subtype	Effects	Receptor blockers	Mode of action
α_1	Vasoconstriction	Phenoxybenzamine	Increase IP3 DAG and calcium
	Pupillary dilatation	Doxazosin	
α_2	Vasoconstriction		Decrease cAMP
β_1	Increased heart rate	Propranolol	Increase cAMP
	Increased cardiac contractility	Atenolol	Increase cAMP
β_2	Bronchial dilatation		
	Increased hepatic glucose output		
β_3	Increase hepatic glucose output		Increase cAMP
	Increase lipolysis		

Circulating catecholamines are very rapidly metabolized and inactivated by an enzyme called carboxy-*O*-methyl transferase (COMT), which is found in most tissues of the body. It converts adrenaline to metadrenaline and noradrenaline to normetadrenaline. These can then be converted by monoamine oxidase to vanillyl-mandelic acid (VMA), which is excreted in the urine. Catecholamines can also be conjugated in the liver. Usually, around 50% of catecholamines are excreted in the met- form with 35% converted to VMA and most of the remaining 15% excreted as conjugates.

Actions of adrenal medullary hormones

These hormones are part of the classical 'fight or flight' neuroendocrine response. Catecholamines activate a group of receptors called 'adrenoceptors' and have a wide range of actions in many different cell and tissue types. Physiologically, their major effects are on the cardiovascular system, causing an increase in heart rate, cardiac contractility and raised blood pressure. They cause both pupillary and bronchial dilatation, and increased glucose production by the liver. They also cause sphincter contraction and muscle relaxation in the gut and the bladder.

The adrenoceptors activated by adrenaline and noradrenaline are classified as either alpha or beta. Different receptors mediate the different effects of catecholamines. See Table 5.1 for an indication of the effects associated with activation of different receptor subtypes, and the drugs that may be used to block these effects. Adrenoceptor blockers are competitive inhibitors of the receptor (i.e. they can be displaced from the receptors by high concentrations of catecholamines). In general adrenaline is more potent than noradrenaline at beta receptors while noradrenaline is

---

Case 5.1 Phaeochromocytoma: 2

Case note: Establishing the diagnosis
What is the cause of Mrs Smith's signs and symptoms?

Mrs Smith had over-secretion of the catecholamines noradrenaline and adrenaline. This is usually the result of a tumour called a phaeochromocytoma.

The overall action of catecholamines is the response to stress ('fight and flight'). The heart beats faster and stronger, and blood pressure and blood sugar levels rise. There is reduced blood flow to non-vital organs, dilatation of the pupils and airways, and increased sweating.

Case 5.1 Phaeochromocytoma: 3

Case note: Treatment

Mrs Smith was treated with an α-adrenoreceptor blocking drug, phenoxybenzamine. A β-adrenoreceptor drug, propranolol, was given a few hours later. The treatment resulted in a steady fall of the blood pressure to 130/80 mmHg.

The likeliest source of high levels of catecholamines in Mrs Smith was a phaeochromocytoma of the adrenal medulla. Therefore, a computed tomographic scan of the abdomen and adrenal glands was carried out, showing a mass in the right adrenal gland. Had the adrenal gland been normal, a tumour might have been found in any of the sympathetic ganglia situated from the base of the skull to the bottom of the pelvis. In Mrs Smith's case, an isotope test was also carried out to confirm that the adrenal mass was a phaeochromocytoma. This scan used a chemical called MIBG ([131]I-*m*-iodobenzylguanidine), which is taken up by catecholamine-producing tissues. This mass took up the radio-isotope MIBG, confirming it to be a phaeochromocytoma.

Several weeks later, and protected by regular treatment with phenoxybenzamine and propranolol, a surgeon removed the right adrenal gland and tumour.

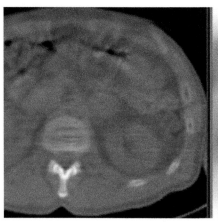
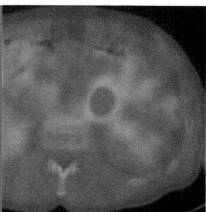

(A)

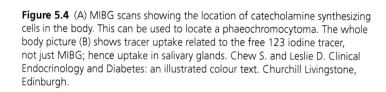

(B)

Figure 5.4 (A) MIBG scans showing the location of catecholamine synthesizing cells in the body. This can be used to locate a phaeochromocytoma. The whole body picture (B) shows tracer uptake related to the free 123 iodine tracer, not just MIBG; hence uptake in salivary glands. Chew S. and Leslie D. Clinical Endocrinology and Diabetes: an illustrated colour text. Churchill Livingstone, Edinburgh.

more potent than adrenaline at alpha receptors. Activation of different receptors can bring about opposing effects, so activation of beta 2 receptors stimulates insulin secretion while activation of alpha 2 receptors inhibits insulin release. Beta adrenoceptors all act by stimulating an increase in cAMP, while alpha adrenoceptors either act through phospholipase C (alpha 1 receptors) or by decreasing cAMP (alpha 2 receptors).

While the adrenal medulla secretes small amounts of dopamine, which circulates in blood, this has no known physiological function. The major functions of dopamine are as a neurotransmitter in the central nervous system, and in the regulation of prolactin secretion (see Ch. 4).

Disorders of the adrenal medulla: phaeochromocytoma

There is no clinical condition arising from an insufficiency of adrenal medullary catecholamines. If both adrenal glands are removed it is necessary only to give cortical steroids as hormone replacement. Sufficient adrenaline and noradrenaline are produced by the rest of the sympathetic nervous system to preserve the 'fight or flight' response.

However, over-secretion of adrenal medullary hormones causes a serious endocrine disorder. Adrenal medullary over-secretion arises as a result of a tumour of the adrenal medulla called a phaeochromocytoma. A phaeochromocytoma can occur in any sympathetic ganglion but is most commonly found in the adrenal medulla. Localization of the tumour is achieved by carrying out an MIBG scan. This marker is taken up by catecholamine-synthesizing cells and provides a reliable means of locating the tumour (Fig. 5.4).

The symptoms of a phaeochromocytoma are like having a fright several times a day. The release of catecholamines occurs episodically over the day, so somebody would experience what felt like a series of panic attacks: increased heart rate, sweating and anxiety. The excess

release of catecholamines also causes an increase in blood pressure which can be life-threatening. This condition is treated by blocking the actions of the catecholamines, as it is not possible to block their synthesis. When treating a phaeochromocytoma it is important to give alpha adrenoceptor blockers before giving beta adrenoceptor blockers. If the beta blockers are started first this reduces the beneficial vasodilator effects of beta receptors and can cause a very dangerous increase in blood pressure. Starting alpha blockers first avoids this. Calcium channel blockers are also used to treat phaeochromocytoma. However, as soon as the patient has had their blood pressure stabilized by drug treatment, the tumour is surgically removed.

Interesting fact

While the catecholamines are the most important products of a phaeochromocytoma, an adrenal medullary tumour can secrete a very wide range of peptides and neurotransmitters including ACTH, growth hormone, calcitonin, somatostatin, neuropeptide Y, erythropoietin and vasoactive intestinal polypeptide (VIP). The potent vasodilatory peptide, adrenomedullin (see Ch. 13), was originally identified in extracts from a phaeochromocytoma.

Familial phaeochromocytoma

About 25% of cases of phaeochromocytoma are familial, in other words inherited due to genetic abnormalities. Although these genetic mutations are rare, they can provide important information about how systems work normally and the variety of ways in which they can go wrong. Table 5.2 shows the five different gene mutations which are known to cause familial phaeochromocytoma and their associated inherited syndromes. Mutations in the succinate dehydrogenase gene are the most likely finding in familial phaeochromocytoma and the SDHB sub-type are particularly important to identify as the tumours are

Table 5.2 Genetic causes of familial phaeochromocytoma

Gene	Protein	Syndrome
Succinate dehydrogenase complex, subunit B (SDHB)	Iron-sulphur protein	Paraganglioma and phaeo syndromes
Succinate dehydrogenase complex, subunit D (SDHD)	CybS (Membrane protein)	Paraganglioma and phaeo syndromes
VHL (Von Hippel Lindau gene)	pVHL9 and pVHL30	Von Hippel Lindau syndrome
RET	Tyrosine kinase receptor	MEN 2a and 2b
NF1	Neurofibromin	Neurofibrinomatosis type 1

MEN, multiple endocrine neoplasia. See Ch. 13.

commonly extra-adrenal and malignant. Because of the increased risk of malignancy, the need to treat associated conditions and the need for longer follow-up, genetic testing for familial phaeochromocytoma is routinely offered to patients presenting with phaeochromocytoma who have a positive family history or who are aged under 50.

Pharmacological uses of hormones of the adrenal medulla

The catecholamines have some highly specialized pharmacological uses. Adrenaline is commonly used in conjunction with a local anaesthetic, particularly in dentistry. The adrenaline causes vasoconstriction and so acts to reduce local blood flow. By doing this, it slows the rate of absorption of the anaesthetic and so prolongs its duration of action.

Adrenaline has an important use in the emergency treatment of acute anaphylaxis. It is carried in the form of an EpiPen, by many people at risk of developing anaphylactic shock as a result of severe allergies. The adrenaline is self-administered by intramuscular injection. Emergency medical teams also use adrenaline intravenously for the treatment of anaphylaxis, severe asthma attacks and for cardiac resuscitation. The effects of injected adrenaline are bronchodilation, vasoconstriction and increased heart rate, so it reverses the catastrophic plunge in blood pressure seen in anaphylaxis, eases breathing in asthma and helps to maintain heart rate in cardiac failure.

Endocrine hypertension

High blood pressure is classified into essential hypertension or secondary hypertension. The cause of essential hypertension is unknown and most patients fall into this category. However, in approximately 10% of patients hypertension is secondary to an underlying cause. Secondary hypertension is classified into renal, endocrine and vascular causes. Endocrine causes of hypertension include hyperaldosteronism (Conn's syndrome), Cushing's syndrome and phaeochromocytoma.

THE ADRENAL GLANDS PART II:
THE ADRENAL CORTEX

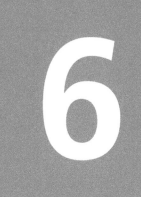

Chapter objectives

After studying this chapter you should be able to:

1. Describe how the adrenal cortex is regulated and explain the principles of negative feedback.

2. Describe how the major adrenocortical hormones are synthesized.

3. Describe the therapeutic uses of glucocorticoids and their unwanted effects.

4. Describe the effects of both under- and over-production of adrenal hormones.

5. Describe the normal development of the adrenal cortex and explain how abnormal development results in disease.

Introduction

The location and general structure of the adrenal gland have been described in the previous chapter, where we looked at the functions of the hormones of the medulla. This chapter concentrates on the hormones of the adrenal cortex, which are less well known than the medullary hormones, but much more important. It is entirely possible to live a healthy life without an adrenal medulla, but if you have no adrenal cortex, then hormone replacement therapy is essential. We shall look at the steroids secreted by the adrenal cortex, consider the effects of both over- and under-production of these hormones and also explore their pharmacological uses.

Structure of the adrenal cortex

The adrenal cortex is the outermost part of the adrenal gland and totally encloses the adrenal medulla (Fig. 6.1). The cells of the adrenal cortex can be divided into three types, arranged in concentric shells or zones. The outermost zone, immediately beneath the connective tissue capsule, is the zona glomerulosa, named after the Latin word for 'ball of wool'. Indeed the cells of this zone are arranged in clusters and, with a little imagination, could be said to resemble balls of wool. This zone is usually only 5–7 cells thick, although this varies with physiological state. Someone who is chronically sodium-deprived has a larger zona glomerulosa than someone with a normal sodium intake.

The middle of the three zones is the zona fasciculata. This is named after the Latin for a 'bundle of sticks'. The cells of this zone are arranged in radial cords, long strings of cells which stretch from the zona glomerulosa towards the medulla. They do look a little bit like bundles of sticks. The third zone, which is next to the adrenal medulla is the zona reticularis. This means 'network' and the cells do appear to form a loose sort of network. All the cells of the adrenal cortex have the characteristic appearance of steroid-secreting cells. They contain lipid droplets and large numbers of mitochondria.

Functionally, the main difference is between the zona glomerulosa and the other two zones. The zona glomerulosa is the only zone that produces the mineralocorticoid, aldosterone. The zona fasciculata and zona reticularis both produce the glucocorticoid, cortisol and the adrenal androgens. In general, the zona fasciculata produces more cortisol and the zona reticularis produces more androgens.

Hormones produced by the adrenal cortex

The adrenal cortex secretes a range of steroid hormones. The most important of these are cortisol (a glucocorticoid) and aldosterone (a mineralocorticoid). Aldosterone is produced exclusively by the cells of the zona glomerulosa, whereas cortisol comes from the zona fasciculata and zona reticularis (Fig. 6.2). These zones also produce very large quantities of dehydroepiandrosterone

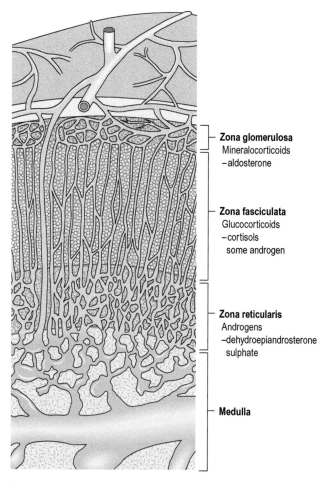

Zona glomerulosa
Mineralocorticoids
–aldosterone

Zona fasciculata
Glucocorticoids
–cortisols
  some androgen

Zona reticularis
Androgens
–dehydroepiandrosterone
  sulphate

Medulla

Figure 6.2 Cross-section through the adrenal gland to show the zonal arrangement of cells, and the major steroid secreted by each zone.

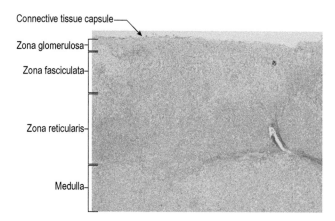

Connective tissue capsule

Zona glomerulosa

Zona fasciculata

Zona reticularis

Medulla

Figure 6.1 Histological section through the adrenal gland showing the general cellular morphology.

(DHEA), a weak androgen that can be converted to both androgens and oestrogens in other tissues of the body. Most of the DHEA is secreted in a sulphated form, as DHEAS. Unlike peptide hormones, the steroids are not stored within the adrenal cells, but instead the gland stores a large amount of cholesterol esters, the substrate for steroid synthesis. These are stored as lipid droplets within the cells, giving the adrenal its classical histological appearance (Fig. 6.4). Normal circulating levels of adrenal hormones are shown in Table 6.1.

Steroid biosynthesis (steroidogenesis)

All adrenal steroids are synthesized from cholesterol by a series of mostly hydroxylation reactions. The pathway of adrenal steroid biosynthesis is shown in Figure 6.5. The enzymes that catalyse steroid hydroxylations are all members of the cytochrome P450 enzyme family encoded by genes of the *CYP* family (Table 6.2). Curiously, these enzymes are not co-localized within the cell, but are located both in mitochondria and in the smooth endoplasmic reticulum. The first reaction of cortisol biosynthesis takes place in the mitochondrion, but the next three reactions, up to the formation of 11-deoxycortisol take place in the smooth endoplasmic reticulum, while the final reaction, the conversion of 11-deoxycortisol to cortisol, again takes place in the mitochondrion. So the intermediate steroids have to be transported around the adrenal cell during their synthesis. Given the lipophilic nature of these intermediate products, it is surprising that they do not simply leak out of the cell. However, this does not happen to any great extent, so the intermediate products on the pathway are not normally secreted in significant quantities, and their presence in the circulation can suggest an adrenal disorder (see Box 1). The major secreted products are highlighted.

It is also quite remarkable that the process of steroidogenesis happens so quickly: increased steroid output by the adrenal is usually seen within two minutes of exposure to ACTH stimulation. The rate-limiting step of steroid biosynthesis is the conversion of cholesterol to pregnenolone, a reaction catalysed by cytochrome P450 side chain cleavage, encoded by *CYP 11A1*. This enzyme is located on the inner mitochondrial membrane of the adrenal cells and it is the rate of transport of cholesterol across from the outer to the inner mitochondrial membrane that limits the rate of steroid biosynthesis. This

---

Case 6.1 Congenital adrenal hyperplasia: 1

Case history

A 4-year-old girl was brought to the paediatric clinic with failure to thrive. The mother reported that her daughter was always thirsty and passed urine frequently. Both height and weight of the child were lower than expected (below the 10th percentile). Pubic hair developed from the age of 3 years and there was an enlarged clitoris with partial fusion of the labial folds (Fig. 6.3). The blood pressure was 70/30 mmHg (normal for a 4-year-old is 90/50 mmHg).

Blood tests were taken:

Serum sodium	127 mmol/L (normal, 135–145 mmol/L)
Serum potassium	5.4 mmol/L (normal, 3.5–6.5 mmol/L)
Serum cortisol	128 nmol/L (normal, 200–600 nmol/L)
Serum adrenocorticotropic hormone	55 ng/L (normal, <50 ng/L)
Lying plasma renin activity	1242 pmol/L/h (normal, 230–1000 pmol/L/h)
Serum 17-hydroxyprogesterone	76 nmol/L (normal before puberty, <3 nmol/L).

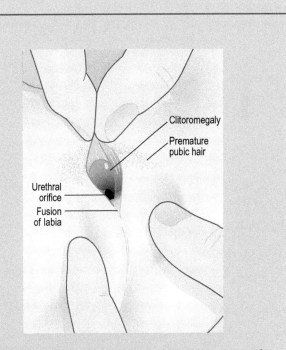

Figure 6.3 Ambiguous genitalia on a baby girl, characteristic of a severe case of congenital adrenal hyperplasia. Note the fused labia and enlarged clitoris. Note also the pubic hair (from Chew S L, Leslie D. 2006. Clinical endocrinology and diabetes: an illustrated colour text. Churchill Livingstone, Edinburgh, with permission).

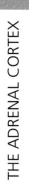

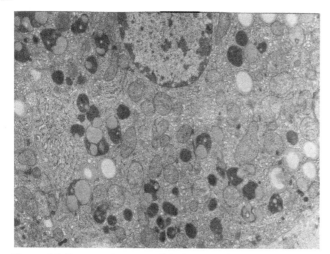

Figure 6.4 Electron microscopy of the human adrenal zona fasciculata, showing lipid droplets and an abundance of mitochondria in the cells (from Belloni A S, Mazzocchi G, Mantero F et al. 1987. J Submicroscopic Cytol 19:657–668, with permission from Editrice Compositori).

Table 6.1   Normal circulating concentrations of the major adrenal steroids in the adult

Steroid	Concentration
Cortisol	
0800 h	220–660 nmol/L
1600 h	50–410 nmol/L
Dehydroepiandrosterone	0.6–70 nmol/L
Dehydroepiandrosterone sulphate	5.4–9.2 μmol/L
Aldosterone	
Recumbent	80–250 pmol/L
Upright	100–831 pmol/L
17α-Hydroxyprogesterone	
Women	1–13 nmol/L
Men	1.5–7.5 nmol/L

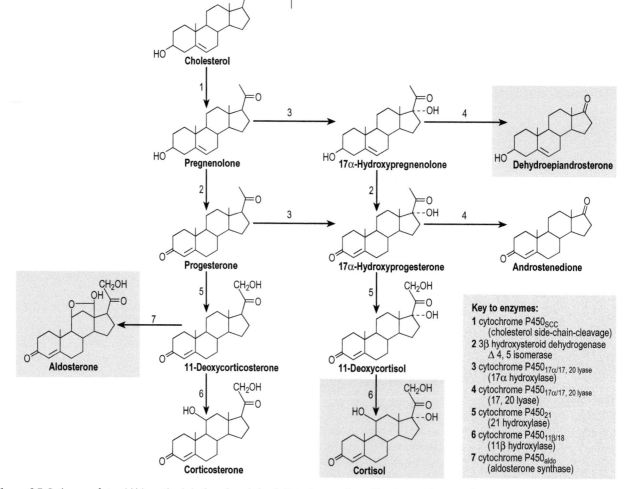

Figure 6.5 Pathways of steroid biosynthesis in the adrenal gland. Note that small modifications to the steroid structure produce significant biological differences. Note also that only seven different enzymes produce this range of adrenal steroids. Most of these enzymes are members of the cytochrome P450 enzyme family.

Table 6.2 Enzymes of steroid biosynthesis, the genes encoding them, the reaction they catalyse and their cellular location

Enzyme	Encoded by	Major reaction catalysed	Cellular location
Cytochrome P450$_{scc}$	CYP 11A1	Cholesterol side-chain cleavage	Mitochondrion
		Conversion of cholesterol to pregnenolone	
3β hydroxysteroid dehydrogenase delta 4,5 isomerase	Not CYP family	Conversion of pregnenolone to progesterone	Smooth ER
Cytochrome P450$_{17alpha/17,20\ lyase}$	CYP17A1	17 hydroxylation of pregnenolone and progesterone	Smooth ER
		Conversion of 17 hydroxypregnenolone to dehydroepiandrosterone	
		Conversion of 17 hydroxyprogesterone to androstenedione	
Cytochrome P450$_{21}$	CYP21A1	Conversion of progesterone to 11 deoxycorticosterone	Smooth ER
		Conversion of 17 hydroxyprogesterone to 11 deoxycortisol	
Cytochrome P450$_{c11B}$	CYP11B1	Conversion of 11 deoxycortisol to cortisol	Mitochondrion
Cytochrome P450$_{c11AS}$ (aldosterone synthase)	CYP11B2	Conversion of 11 deoxycorticosterone to aldosterone	Mitochondrion
17β hydroxysteroid dehydrogenase	Not CYP family	Conversion of androstenedione to testosterone	Smooth ER
Cytochrome P450$_{arom}$	CYP19A	Aromatization of testosterone to 17β oestradiol	Smooth ER

transfer of cholesterol is complex but one protein has been shown to be essential for this to occur. Steroidogenic acute regulatory protein, termed StAR protein, is a rapidly turned-over protein in most steroid-producing cells. When the cell is stimulated by a trophic hormone, cAMP is produced which activates PKA and causes the phosphorylation and activation of StAR. In the absence of functional StAR protein, the adrenals are not able to synthesize steroid hormones. This causes a condition called lipoid adrenal hyperplasia, because the cells of the adrenal cortex become greatly enlarged and filled with lipid droplets containing cholesterol which cannot be used for steroid synthesis because it cannot get across the mitochondrial membrane.

Cholesterol

Cholesterol is the essential starting point for all pathways of steroid synthesis. The source of cholesterol for steroid biosynthesis is mostly from the intracellular lipid droplets. When ACTH binds to receptors on the adrenal cell, the cAMP that this generates causes a number of intracellular changes. StAR protein is phosphorylated as we have seen. An enzyme called cholesterol ester hydrolase is also activated. This enzyme liberates cholesterol from the lipid stores within the cells and this is the cholesterol that is used for steroidogenesis. But where do the lipid droplets come from?

Cholesterol can be made 'de novo' (from scratch) within adrenal cells by the actions of an enzyme called

HMG-CoA reductase. It can also be taken up by adrenal cells in the form of low density lipoproteins (LDL). There is a specific receptor-mediated process of LDL uptake in adrenal cells. ACTH stimulates both of these processes. In human adrenals, if there is a steady supply of LDL in plasma this is the preferred source of cholesterol and de novo synthesis rates are very low.

Defects of steroid biosynthesis

A deficiency of any of the enzymes involved in steroid biosynthesis will cause a decrease in products downstream of the enzyme and an increase in precursors upstream. Such an enzyme deficiency causes a condition called congenital adrenal hyperplasia, so called because the adrenal gland increases in size as the body tries to increase production of adrenal hormones. The plasma concentration of cortisol is insufficient to suppress ACTH and so the adrenal is exposed to elevated ACTH concentrations. The commonest adrenal enzyme deficiency (approximately 90% of cases) affects 21-hydroxylase, which is encoded by the gene CYP21. This enzyme converts progesterone to 11-deoxycorticosterone, and converts 17-hydroxyprogesterone to 11-deoxycortisol (Fig. 6.5). There is, therefore, very low production of both aldosterone and cortisol in patients with 21-hydroxylase (CYP21) mutations. The progesterone and 17-hydroxyprogesterone that accumulate are metabolized via the alternative pathway into androgens (Fig. 6.6).

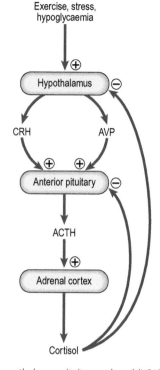

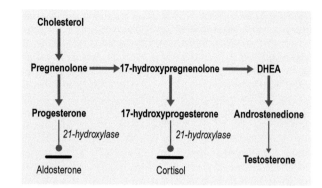

Figure 6.6 The commonest enzyme deficiency causing congenital adrenal hyperplasia is a defect in 21-hydroxylase, which is a key enzyme in the production of both aldosterone and cortisol. It is not required for androgen biosynthesis, however, so the steroid precursors that accumulate are converted into adrenal androgens.

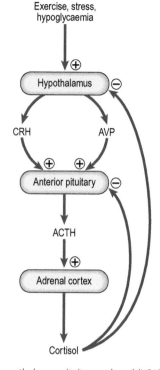

Figure 6.7 The hypothalamo–pituitary–adrenal (HPA) axis. Activity of this axis is stimulated by stress, hypoglycaemia and exercise. This stimulus causes a release of both corticotropin releasing hormone (CRH) and arginine vasopressin (AVP) from the hypothalamus. These two hormones act together on the corticotroph cells of the pituitary to stimulate adrenocorticotropin (ACTH) release. ACTH acts on the adrenal cortex to stimulate the release of cortisol which, in addition to its other actions, exerts a negative feedback effect on both the hypothalamus and pituitary to decrease activity of the HPA axis.

Case 6.1	Congenital adrenal hyperplasia: 2

Case note: Establishing the diagnosis

If you look back at the case history box, what do the levels of serum cortisol and serum 17-hydroxyprogesterone suggest? There is a low serum cortisol level, which might indicate primary adrenocortical failure, but there is a raised serum level of 17-hydroxyprogesterone, which is synthesized in the adrenal cortex, so this cannot be a case of failure of the adrenal cortex. This pattern is characteristic of an error in the cortisol production pathway (Figs 6.5, 6.6), a condition called congenital adrenal hyperplasia. In 90% of cases, this is due to a defect in the gene for the 21-hydroxylase enzyme. This gene defect results in seriously impaired cortisol secretion, but some cortisol is still made. The block in cortisol production results in an accumulation of precursors such as 17-hydroxyprogesterone. The precursors then spill over to make adrenal androgens such as DHEA and androstenedione.

Regulation of steroid production

Cortisol: the hypothalamo–pituitary–adrenal axis

Cortisol is produced mainly by the cells of the zona fasciculata, with smaller amounts coming from the zona reticularis. Cortisol production is regulated by adrenocorticotropic hormone (ACTH), which, in turn, is regulated by corticotropin releasing hormone (CRH) and arginine vasopressin (AVP) secreted by the hypothalamus (see Ch. 3). CRH and AVP have synergistic actions on the corticotroph cells of the anterior pituitary. This means that the actions of the two hormones working together is greater than the sum of their individual effects. It is not well understood how they achieve that but we do know that they both activate different intracellular pathways. Both

CRH and AVP act through specific G-protein coupled receptors on corticotroph cells. The CRH receptors are linked to cyclic AMP generation while the AVP receptors are linked to intracellular calcium signalling.

Cortisol has negative feedback effects both at the level of the hypothalamus, inhibiting CRH and AVP secretion, and the pituitary, inhibiting ACTH secretion. This is the hypothalamo–pituitary–adrenal (HPA) axis (Fig. 6.7). There is a diurnal variation in ACTH production and secretion, and therefore in serum cortisol concentrations, with a peak at 0600–0900 hours (Fig. 6.8). Serum cortisol is therefore usually sampled at 0900 hours. The HPA axis is also stimulated by stress—both by physiological stressors, such as cold exposure, infection, hypoglycaemia and exercise, and also by psychological stressors, such as exams!

The actions of ACTH (Fig. 6.9)

Adrenocorticotropin has a range of effects on the adrenal gland, over a time course of a few seconds to several days. The most immediate effect of ACTH is to cause an increase in blood flow through the adrenal gland. This increases the rate of delivery of oxygen to the

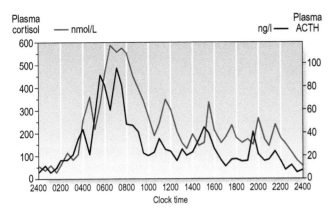

Figure 6.8 Activity of the HPA axis is subject to diurnal variation, with a peak of activity around 0600 hours and a nadir around midnight. Note that the increase in ACTH levels precedes the rise in cortisol. Note also that there are secretory peaks during the day, when the axis is stimulated by other inputs (Fig. 6.7).

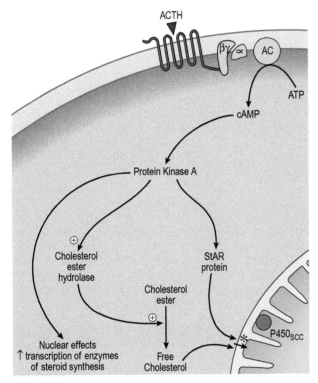

Figure 6.9 Actions of ACTH on the adrenal cell. ACTH binds to a cell surface receptor which is coupled, via a G-protein, to adenylyl cyclase. The cAMP produced activates protein kinase A which phosphorylates both cholesterol ester hydrolase and StAR protein, which respectively liberate cholesterol and transport it across the mitochondrial membrane to initiate steroid synthesis.

gland: steroid synthesis is a highly oxygen-dependent process. Within minutes, there is an increase in steroid secretion and over hours and days ACTH causes an increase in levels of expression of the steroidogenic enzymes and an increase in cellular size. Prolonged high

levels of ACTH secretion cause an increase in the size of the adrenal gland, but it is probably not ACTH itself, but a peptide that is co-secreted with ACTH, that causes the increase in adrenal size.

At the cellular level, ACTH binds to specific receptors in the plasma membrane and causes an increase in intracellular cyclic adenosine monophosphate (cAMP) production. The ACTH receptor is also known as the melanocortin-2 receptor, and belongs to a family of similar receptors. The major result of the action of ACTH is to increase the conversion of cholesterol to pregnenolone, which is the rate-limiting step of steroidogenesis. ACTH achieves this effect in several ways: by increasing the availability of cholesterol within the cell, by increasing the rate of cholesterol uptake into the cell through HDL and LDL receptors and by increasing the rate of cholesterol delivery to the enzyme, rather than by affecting enzyme activity directly. This last effect is achieved by the activation of StAR protein and is the rate-limiting step.

Because cortisol production is subject to negative feedback regulation (see Ch. 1), decreased cortisol production results in increased ACTH secretion in an attempt to restore cortisol levels. ACTH acts both to increase steroid synthesis and to maintain the size and function of the adrenal gland. When cortisol synthesis is impaired, serum ACTH levels can increase significantly, leading to increased adrenal size, called adrenal hyperplasia.

Case 6.1 Congenital adrenal hyperplasia: 3

Clinical note: Explanation of plasma ACTH result

Cortisol regulates ACTH secretion by exerting a negative feedback effect on both the hypothalamus and pituitary, so low cortisol levels result in increased ACTH secretion. The effect of ACTH is to drive production of steroid precursors prior to the enzyme defect and induce growth (hyperplasia) of the adrenal cortices.

Aldosterone: the renin–angiotensin system

Aldosterone is produced exclusively by the cells of the zona glomerulosa. Aldosterone production is regulated principally by the renin–angiotensin system (Fig. 6.10). The renin–angiotensin system is an example of a cascade of protein cleavage steps. Another example (outside the endocrine system) is the clotting cascade. When reduced renal perfusion or a low plasma sodium concentration is detected, the juxtaglomerular cells of the kidney release renin into the circulation. Renin is a proteolytic enzyme that cleaves a large protein secreted by the liver, angiotensinogen, to produce angiotensin I, a small peptide. Angiotensin I circulates in the blood and is cleaved by another enzyme, termed angiotensin converting enzyme

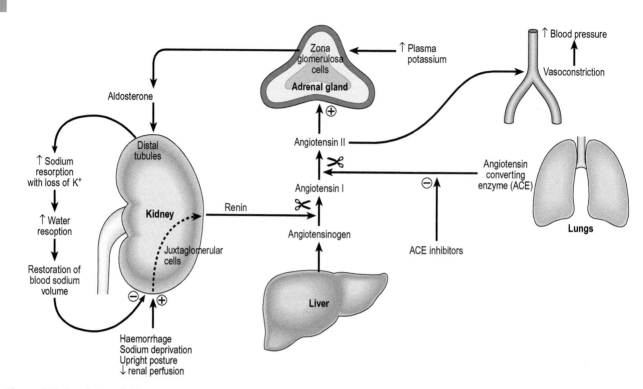

Figure 6.10 Regulation of aldosterone secretion. Aldosterone has a key role in the maintenance of plasma sodium concentrations and is regulated by the renin–angiotensin system. Briefly, starting at the kidneys, renin is released in response to low renal perfusion (may result from blood loss or postural hypotension) or low plasma sodium ion concentration. Renin is a proteolytic enzyme that cleaves angiotensinogen (a large protein secreted by the liver) to release angiotensin I. The angiotensin I is in turn cleaved by angiotensin converting enzyme (ACE), which is located on the luminal surface of vascular endothelial cells, particularly in the lung. The action of ACE generates angiotensin II, which is both a potent vasoconstrictor and the major stimulus to aldosterone secretion. Aldosterone acts on the distal tubules of the kidney, promoting sodium resorption which leads to restoration of blood volume and sodium concentration.

(ACE) to produce angiotensin II. Angiotensin II stimulates aldosterone secretion by binding to receptors in the plasma membrane of zona glomerulosa cells, and increasing phosphatidylinositol turnover (see Ch. 2).

Interesting fact

Angiotensin II is a potent vasoconstrictor in addition to its effects on aldosterone secretion. A first-line treatment for hypertension is an ACE inhibitor, which blocks the formation of angiotensin II. Examples of ACE inhibitors include enalapril, lisinopril and perindopril.

DHEA/S

The adrenal androgens, dehydroepiandrosterone (DHEA) and its sulphated form (DHEAS), are, by mass, the major products of the human adrenal cortex. They are not produced in significant quantities in other species. The zona reticularis is the main site of production of adrenal androgens. Although ACTH stimulates adrenal androgen secretion, this is not the whole story as there are many situations in which cortisol and DHEA production are dissociated. This is particularly so in ageing, when DHEA

secretion declines significantly while cortisol remains relatively constant through life. In the 1970s and early 1980s there was much research effort directed to finding an 'adrenal androgen stimulating hormone', which has still not been found.

Transport of steroid hormones in blood

Steroid hormones are not naturally very soluble in aqueous solutions such as blood. Many steroid hormones therefore have specific binding proteins, which act to increase their solubility and decrease their metabolism. About 95% of circulating cortisol is bound to plasma proteins, mostly to the specific cortisol binding globulin (CBG), and the rest to albumin. Aldosterone does not have a specific binding protein and is transported in blood with around 60% weakly bound to CBG and plasma albumin.

Actions of adrenal steroids

The major hormonal products of the adrenal cortex are cortisol, aldosterone and adrenal androgens.

Physiological actions of cortisol

The effects of cortisol and similar hormones are termed 'glucocorticoid' because, although cortisol has many actions, its effects on glucose homeostasis were the first to be understood. The term glucocorticoid is now used to refer more properly to hormones that bind to the intracellular glucocorticoid receptor through which cortisol exerts its various effects.

Cortisol has a wide range of effects on glucose homeostasis that oppose, but are generally less important than, the effects of insulin. The overall effects of cortisol on metabolism are to maintain blood glucose levels and liver glycogen stores when the body is in the fasting state. Cortisol stimulates protein catabolism in muscle, lipolysis in adipose tissue, and both gluconeogenesis (conversion of non-glucose molecules into new glucose) and glycogenolysis (breakdown of glycogen to release glucose) in the liver (Box 6.1).

Cortisol is able to counteract many of the components of the inflammatory response to tissue injury. It does this by inhibiting the production or action of some of the chemical mediators of inflammation such as histamine, prostaglandins and leukotrienes. Similarly, although cortisol is needed for normal B-lymphocyte function, higher levels of cortisol suppress many aspects of the immune response. Under these conditions cortisol decreases both the number and the effectiveness of T and B lymphocytes. It is likely that the physiological role of cortisol as an anti-inflammatory and immunosuppressant agent is to prevent damage due to excess activity of the inflammatory and immune systems. Both of these effects are utilized therapeutically and are discussed below.

Physiological levels of cortisol are needed for a normal vascular response to noradrenaline. In the absence of cortisol the vasculature is much less responsive to noradrenaline, generally resulting in hypotension. In addition to its negative feedback effects on CRH and ACTH, it is likely that cortisol has important actions on the brain, which are still poorly understood. Glucocorticoid receptors are present throughout the cerebral cortex and are particularly concentrated in the limbic system, suggesting that cortisol may affect mood, learning and memory.

Cortisol is considered to be a stress hormone because its production is increased in response to a variety of physical and psychological stressors. There is a paradox here though. Cortisol is an essential part of the body's response to stress and in the absence of cortisol even moderate stresses can be fatal. On the other hand, cortisol appears to have a role in both damping down potentially damaging effects and in terminating the stress response.

Physiological actions of aldosterone

The actions of aldosterone (Fig. 6.10) are termed 'mineralocorticoid effects' because these actions are on electrolyte balance. Aldosterone acts on the distal convoluted tubule of the kidney nephron and increases sodium reabsorption in exchange for potassium. It brings about this effect by increasing the number of sodium transporter proteins in the nephron. In the kidney, water usually follows the movement of sodium, so aldosterone exerts an anti-diuretic effect.

Like other steroid hormones, aldosterone binds to intracellular receptors which are able to interact with DNA to alter the rate of transcription of specific genes (see Ch. 2). The mineralocorticoid receptor has the same affinity for both aldosterone and cortisol, and so binds both hormones equally well. As the concentration of cortisol in blood exceeds that of aldosterone by around 1000-fold it might be predicted that the receptor would always be occupied by cortisol and that aldosterone would be a redundant hormone. The mineralocorticoid receptor does manage to specifically bind aldosterone; it does this by being located together with an enzyme that removes cortisol from the environment of the receptor, thus protecting the receptor from circulating cortisol. The enzyme is 11β-hydroxysteroid dehydrogenase, which converts cortisol to the inactive cortisone, and is found in all mineralocorticoid target tissues (Fig. 6.11).

Case 6.1 — Congenital adrenal hyperplasia: 4

Case note: Salt wasting

In the clinical case, do you think that serum aldosterone levels would be low, normal or high, given the sodium and potassium measurements?

It is likely that plasma aldosterone levels will be low. The high serum potassium and low serum sodium levels are symptoms of mineralocorticoid deficiency. Normally aldosterone acts to raise serum sodium and decrease serum potassium levels, so lack of aldosterone results in low serum sodium and high serum potassium levels. The raised plasma renin activity is a response to the mineralocorticoid deficiency.

The failure to conserve urinary sodium is called 'salt wasting', and is associated with a diuresis, causing polyuria and thirst.

Box 6.1 Effects of glucocorticoids

Metabolic effects
- Stimulate mobilization of glucose in liver (glycogenolysis and gluconeogenesis)
- Stimulate breakdown of fats and proteins
- Increase plasma concentrations of glucose, fatty acids and amino acids

Cardiovascular effects
- Maintain blood volume: increased glucose concentration draws water into blood compartment
- Maintain vascular responsiveness to catecholamines

Other effects
- Anti-inflammatory: inhibit prostaglandin synthesis
- Immunosuppressive.

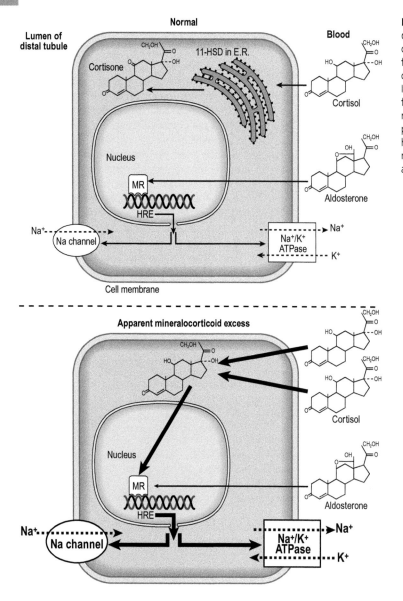

Figure 6.11 Role of 11-beta hydroxysteroid dehydrogenase in mineralocorticoid action. Under normal conditions the mineralocorticoid receptor is protected from high levels of circulating cortisol by the presence of the enzyme 11-beta hydroxysteroid dehydrogenase. In apparent mineralocorticoid excess, this enzyme is not functional and so cortisol binds to the mineralocorticoid receptor and stimulates the production of sodium channel proteins leading to the re-absorption of sodium at a higher rate than is required for normal salt balance. This results is in a condition of high sodium and low potassium, accompanied by hypertension.

Interesting fact

A clinical condition, apparent mineralocorticoid excess (AME), may be caused by eating excessive quantities of liquorice. It was discovered that liquorice contains glycyrrhetinic acid, an inhibitor of 11β-hydroxysteroid dehydrogenase. The liquorice removes the protection given by 11 beta hydroxysteroid dehydrogenase to the mineralocorticoid receptor, which is then swamped by circulating cortisol (Fig. 6.11). The main symptoms of AME are hypertension with low serum potassium levels.

Actions of adrenal androgens

The effects of adrenal androgens are generally considered to be significant only in disease states where they are produced in excessive quantities. Under these conditions the adrenal androgens, which are only weakly androgenic compared with testosterone, can have significant virilizing

Case 6.1 Congenital adrenal hyperplasia: 5

Case note: Revisiting symptoms and signs

As this child is unable to produce normal physiological concentrations of cortisol and aldosterone she is suffering from symptoms of both glucocorticoid and mineralocorticoid deficiency. She is therefore generally unwell, likely to be hypotensive, and will be unable to tolerate stress. Between feeds her blood glucose level is likely to fall. She is also unable to conserve sodium and has 'salt wasting'. Not all cases of congenital adrenal hyperplasia are associated with salt wasting, as some other adrenal hormones, notably 11-deoxycorticosterone, have mineralocorticoid activity. A deficiency of the 11-hydroxylase enzyme will therefore still cause congenital adrenal hyperplasia, but without the symptom of salt wasting.

Case 6.1 Congenital adrenal hyperplasia: 6

Case note: Precocious puberty

In the clinical case, why has the child developed an enlarged clitoris and pubic hair? The presence of pubic hair indicates that this child has developed precocious puberty, which may result from over-production of sex steroids, such as 17-hydroxyprogesterone. The enlarged clitoris is a result of the excess adrenal androgen production, causing abnormal genital development in female babies.

Interesting fact

Although DHEA is conventionally regarded simply as a weak androgen, there is some evidence that it may be more significant than this. Production declines markedly throughout adult life, unlike the other adrenal steroids, and the circulating DHEA concentration is much lower in a variety of disease states. For these reasons DHEA has become a popular anti-ageing remedy, although there is little evidence that taking this steroid has any effect at all on the normal ageing process.

Disorders of adrenal steroids

Congenital adrenal hyperplasia (CAH)

This disorder is an example of an inborn error of metabolism, in which there is a deficiency of one of the enzymes of steroid biosynthesis. This occurs as a result of a gene mutation, most commonly of CYP21, the gene encoding 21-hydroxylase (Fig. 6.6). As a result of the enzyme insufficiency there is inadequate secretion of glucocorticoids and mineralocorticoids, and excess secretion of adrenal androgens. Severe forms of CAH are usually detected at birth in girls because of the ambiguous genitalia (see Case history), but can be more difficult to diagnose in boys. The main symptom of CAH in babies is a general 'failure to thrive'.

effects. This may result in the development of ambiguous genitalia in female infants with an adrenal disorder, and in hirsutism and acne in women with excess adrenal androgen production. Adrenal androgens may be converted to oestrogens by the action of aromatase, principally in adipose tissue, providing the only source of oestrogens in postmenopausal women. For this reason, there was, briefly in the early 20th century, a trend for removing the adrenal glands in postmenopausal women with a hormone-dependent cancer, such as breast cancer.

Case 6.1 Congenital adrenal hyperplasia: 7

Case note: Treatment and follow-up

The principle of treatment is to give sufficient glucocorticoid to suppress ACTH secretion, so that adrenal androgen production falls within the normal range. The patient will also need fludrocortisone (a synthetic mineralocorticoid).

The patient was treated with hydrocortisone, 5 mg daily in the morning. She underwent surgery to divide the fused labia. When aged 14 years, the hydrocortisone was increased to 10 mg daily in the morning to keep pace with her growth. At age 24 years she was referred for genetic counselling as she was now keen to start a family.

What problems do you anticipate and how may these be managed?

Congenital adrenal hyperplasia is one of the commonest autosomal recessive genetic diseases. Thus, patients with this form of congenital adrenal hyperplasia have mutations or deletions of both copies (alleles) of the 21-hydroxylase gene. In this case the fetus will be a carrier of a mutated allele inherited from the mother. A fetus will have congenital adrenal hyperplasia only if the father is also a carrier of a mutated allele and this is inherited by the fetus. Carriers of mutations in the 21-hydroxylase gene may be found commonly in some populations, and the risk is increased by consanguinity. Before pregnancy is recommended, the partner can be offered a genetic test for common mutations of the gene. If this is not possible or is refused, a biopsy of the placenta (chorionic biopsy) can be performed in the early weeks of pregnancy to test whether the fetus is female. Affected female babies can have severely virilized external genitalia and this can be prevented by steroid treatment (in the form of dexamethasone, which crosses the placenta). Potentially affected babies are tested by measuring the 17-hydroxyprogesterone level in the cord blood at birth, because they are at risk of salt wasting and circulatory collapse.

Glucocorticoid excess

Cushing's syndrome is the term for any disorder of glucocorticoid excess. It is named after Harvey Cushing (1868–1939), an American neurosurgeon who studied the pituitary gland. There are several possible causes of Cushing's syndrome (Box 6.2). The symptoms of glucocorticoid excess produce a marked change in the appearance of a person, who classically develops a rounded 'moon face' with truncal obesity and muscle wasting in the arms and legs. The skin becomes thinned, with striae developing, and an increased tendency to bruising (Fig. 6.12).

In addition to the alterations in physical appearance, hypercortisolaemia can also result in hypertension, osteoporosis and diabetes mellitus. Wound healing is impaired and there is an increased risk of infection as the immune system is suppressed. There are significant mood

Case 6.2 Cushing's syndrome: 1

Case history

Mr Jones, a 38-year-old divorced warehouse manager, has suffered from severe asthma since childhood. He has been taking prednisolone, 30 mg orally daily, for the past 18 months. He had become worried after reading about the side-effects of steroids and had stopped taking the steroid tablets 3 weeks previously. He was particularly worried about his beer belly, which looked very fat compared with his skinny arms and legs. His sister visited and found him looking very unwell, having been on a long run the day before, as the start of his new exercise regime. She immediately called in the general practitioner. On arrival, the GP found Mr Jones to be pale and suffering from nausea and vomiting. Blood pressure was 80/40 mmHg when lying and unrecordable on standing. An ambulance was called and Mr Jones was rushed to the nearest A&E department. On arrival, blood was taken and the following plasma concentrations of urea and electrolytes (Us and Es) were obtained:

Serum sodium	127 mmol/L (normal range 136–146 mmol/L)
Serum potassium	6.0 mmol/L (normal range 3.5–5.1 mmol/L)
Serum urea	12.2 mmol/l (normal range 2.5–4 mmol/L)

The next morning blood was taken at 0900 h and the following concentrations were obtained:

Serum cortisol	<50 nmol/L (normal range 200–600 nmol/L)
Serum ACTH	<2 ng/L (normal range 10–50 ng/L)

Mr Jones was treated with intravenous fluids and steroids, and made a rapid recovery. Before discharge, the side-effects of steroids were discussed and Mr Jones was counselled about the dangers of stopping steroids abruptly.

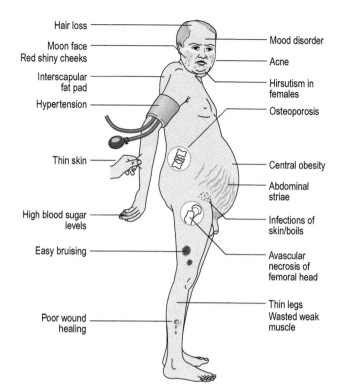

Figure 6.12 Major features of Cushing's syndrome. Acne, baldness and hirsutism are features of Cushing's syndrome which is due to overactive adrenal glands, as these symptoms result from excess production of adrenal androgens.

Box 6.2 Causes of Cushing's syndrome in order of frequency

1. Exogenous corticosteroid administration
2. Cushing's disease (hypersecretion of ACTH from the pituitary)
3. Adrenal adenoma
4. Ectopic ACTH production (e.g. from small cell carcinoma).

disorders associated with Cushing's syndrome. If the disorder is caused by exogenous administration of steroid, this is most commonly associated with elation, whereas excess endogenous steroid is most commonly associated with depression.

Investigations of glucocorticoid excess

Investigations into glucocorticoid excess are based on an assessment of the feedback of the HPA axis. The first step is to measure serum levels of cortisol and ACTH. In cases where Cushing's syndrome is caused by exogenous steroids, such as prednisolone, the serum cortisol and ACTH will be undetectable (note that prednisolone is not usually significantly detected by most cortisol assays). In contrast, cortisol levels may be obviously high in patients

Case 6.2 Cushing's syndrome: 2

Case note: Diagnosis

What was the cause of Mr Jones' change in body shape? Mr Jones had probably developed Cushing's syndrome as a result of the high dose of prednisolone he was taking to control his asthma. The beer belly and skinny arms and legs he had noticed were truncal obesity and peripheral wasting.

with an excess of endogenous cortisol. A high serum cortisol with a low ACTH level suggests an adrenocortical tumour secreting cortisol. A high serum cortisol with a detectable serum ACTH level suggests a tumour over-secreting ACTH. ACTH-secreting tumours are usually pituitary adenomas and the condition is then called Cushing's disease.

The usual principle of endocrinology is to try to suppress a hormone that is thought to be abnormally increased in concentration. In Cushing's syndrome, the commonest test is a dexamethasone suppression test. Dexamethasone is not detected in the blood by the cortisol assay. In a healthy person, intake of dexamethasone at specific doses and times will lead to a suppression of the HPA axis and an undetectable or very low serum cortisol level. If a tumour is over-secreting ACTH or cortisol, the serum cortisol will fail to suppress completely with dexamethasone.

Computed tomography and magnetic resonance imaging are often needed to locate tumours that are over-secreting ACTH or cortisol.

Interesting fact

In the days before pituitary microsurgery became routine, Cushing's disease (ACTH secreting tumour of the pituitary) was treated by surgical removal of the adrenal glands. This removed the source of the steroids, but left the patient with high concentrations of ACTH in their circulation. ACTH is very closely related to the family of peptide hormones, the melanotropins, that cause colour change in reptiles, and it binds to one of the family of melanotropin receptors. When ACTH circulates at very high concentrations, it affects the melanocytes in human skin, causing a characteristic hyperpigmentation (skin darkening). This is called Nelson's syndrome.

Mineralocorticoid excess (Conn's syndrome)

This is a relatively rare disorder, characterized by hypertension and hypokalaemia. It may be caused by an aldosterone-secreting adrenal adenoma, but idiopathic (i.e. of unknown cause) hyperaldosteronism is also seen. Tumours are usually small and may be removed surgically. The idiopathic disorder is treated with an aldosterone receptor blocker, such as spironolactone.

Adrenal insufficiency

Primary adrenal insufficiency is a failure of the adrenal glands to secrete sufficient amounts of glucocorticoid in response to stimulation. It is also known as Addison's disease, named after Thomas Addison (1793–1860), the English physician who originally classified the disorder. It is usually a disease of slow onset, involving the gradual destruction of adrenal tissue, often by autoimmune disease, or by human immunodeficiency virus (HIV) infection or tuberculosis. A significant cause of acute adrenal insufficiency is the sudden, unplanned withdrawal of systemic glucocorticoid therapy. The HPA axis is suppressed by glucocorticoid therapy and it takes a few weeks or even months for the axis to fully recover. Sudden withdrawal of treatment with glucocorticoids,

Box 6.3 Signs and symptoms of acute adrenal insufficiency

- Weakness, fatigue, lethargy
- Dehydration, hypotension
- Nausea and vomiting
- Hyponatraemia, hyperkalaemia.

Case 6.2 | Cushing's syndrome: 3

Explanation of clinical presentation

What is the explanation for Mr Jones' clinical presentation? Mr Jones clearly has acute adrenal insufficiency following the abrupt cessation of his steroid therapy. The acute crisis was probably precipitated by the exercise he had taken on the previous day. Although his potassium level was within the normal range, the increased concentration of urea, indicating dehydration, together with the hyponatraemia, point strongly to adrenal insufficiency.

such as prednisolone, can be fatal, so patients taking this therapy carry a steroid card (see below). The ability of the HPA axis to adapt to loss of tissue is remarkable, and up to 90% of the adrenal cortex can be destroyed before symptoms are seen. However, when the person is exposed to stress, the adrenal cannot respond appropriately and the symptoms of a hypoadrenal crisis develop—*acute adrenal insufficiency* (Box 6.3).

Pharmacological uses of glucocorticoids

The anti-inflammatory and immunosuppressive actions of glucocorticoids are exploited therapeutically to treat many different disorders. A wide range of synthetic glucocorticoids is available (Table 6.3). Prednisolone is an example of a synthetic steroid with mainly glucocorticoid actions, so that it acts rather like cortisol. It is often used as an anti-inflammatory agent and is used most widely as a topical preparation for inflammatory skin disorders, or as an inhaled preparation in the prophylaxis of asthma. When used in these forms the risk of adverse effects is minimized. Glucocorticoids are also used systemically to treat inflammatory diseases, such as systemic lupus erythematosus. There is a significant risk of developing Cushing's syndrome, and of long-term suppression of the HPA axis. All currently available glucocorticoids, except dexamethasone and the closely-related betamethasone, have some mineralocorticoid activity (Table 6.3), and so cause sodium and water retention. Many of the synthetic steroids have very long plasma half-lives (Table 6.3) which can be advantageous in that frequent administration is not needed, but has the disadvantage that they persist in the body and increase the risk of adverse effects.

Table 6.3 Glucocorticoid potencies of some of the commonly used synthetic and natural corticosteroids, their mineralocorticoid potency and duration of action

Steroid	Glucocorticoid potency	Mineralocorticoid potency	Half-life in plasma (h)
Cortisol (hydrocortisone)	1	1	8
Prednisolone	4	0.8	≈24
Methylprednisolone	7	0.5	≈30
Dexamethasone	25–75	0	≈48
Betamethasone	30	0	≈48
Aldosterone	0.3	200–1000	
Fludrocortisone acetate	15	200	
Deoxycorticosterone	0	20	

Case 6.2 Cushing's syndrome: 4

Case note: Cause of cortisol and ACTH results

One of the major side-effects of glucocorticoid therapy is long-term suppression of the HPA axis. When therapy is suddenly discontinued there is a risk of developing the symptoms of adrenal insufficiency.

Interesting fact

Cortisol is the naturally occurring hormone secreted by the adrenal gland. Cortisol is called hydrocortisone when it is used therapeutically. Both names refer to exactly the same substance.

Steroid treatment card

When patients start a long course of oral glucocorticoid therapy they are given a steroid card (Fig. 6.13) to carry, which details the medication they are taking. Its purpose is mainly to inform doctors who may treat the patient in the event of sudden illness or accident, and so prevent problems of adrenal insufficiency. It also reminds patients of the need to take their medication regularly.

Case 6.2 Cushing's syndrome: 5

Case note

How could the GP have helped prevent Mr Jones' illness? If Mr Jones had been given a steroid treatment card, he would probably have been more aware of the dangers of stopping his prednisolone without seeking medical advice.

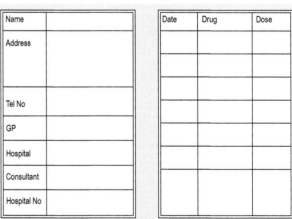

Figure 6.13 Steroid treatment card. All patients receiving treatment with oral glucocorticoids should be given a steroid treatment card. It is designed to ensure that the patient continues to receive an appropriate level of medication if they are in an accident or undergoing surgery, for example.

THE THYROID GLAND

7

Chapter objectives

After studying this chapter you should be able to:

1. Describe the structure of the thyroid glands.

2. Describe how thyroid function is regulated and explain the principles of negative feedback.

3. Describe how thyroid hormones are synthesized and explain the significance of peripheral metabolism of thyroxine.

4. Describe the physiological actions of thyroid hormones.

5. Describe the effects of both under- and over-production of thyroid hormones.

Introduction

The thyroid gland is located in the neck and is about the shape and size of a bow-tie (Fig. 7.1). The name is derived from the Greek word for 'shield', because the shape of the normal thyroid gland resembles a type of bi-lobed shield. The correct functioning of the thyroid gland depends on a supply of iodine in the diet as the hormones it produces are a modified amino acid containing three (T3) or four (T4) iodine atoms. Although the major product of the thyroid gland is T4 (thyroxine), it is T3 which is the more active hormone. Most T3 is produced by peripheral conversion from T4. The thyroid gland has an important role in regulating metabolism and body weight, and thyroid hormones also play an important role in development. Both excess and insufficiency of thyroid hormones results in disease.

Case 7.1 Weight loss: 1

Case history

Mr Smith was a 65-year-old man who attended his general practice because of palpitations, sweating and weight loss, despite a good appetite. The symptoms had been present for about 12 months, but began slowly and insidiously. He described the palpitations as a rapid and irregular beating of the heart in episodes that lasted from several minutes for up to several hours. The sweating occurred with the slightest exercise and was severe enough to drench his bedclothes at night. His weight had fallen from 75 to 63 kg, despite the fact that his appetite and food intake had increased. His wife complained that he was increasingly irritable and had mood swings.

His medical history was negative and there was no use of medication. On direct questioning, Mr Smith admitted to an increased looseness of stools, which were passed twice a day.

On examination, Mr Smith looked well but thin. There was a fine tremor of the hands, which felt hot and sweaty. The pulse was 120 b.p.m. and irregular. There was a mass in the neck (see Fig. 7.2) that rose on swallowing and was firm and nodular. The mass extended behind the notch in the sternum. There was an obvious swelling of both breasts.

Mr Smith's case raises five questions:

1. What is the diagnosis?
2. Why is knowledge of anatomy essential in his management?
3. What is the aetiology and pathogenesis of the disease?
4. What tests should be requested and how should they be interpreted?
5. What are the mechanisms for his symptoms?

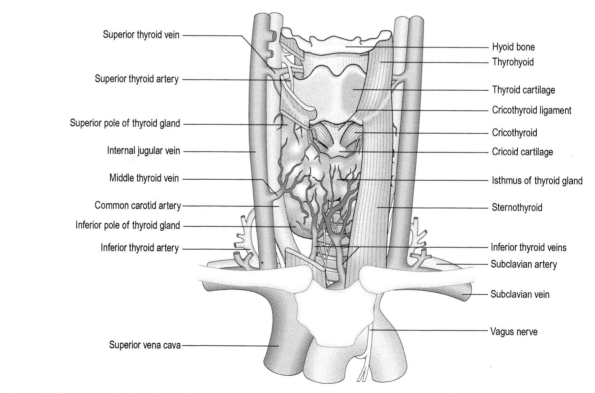

Figure 7.1 Anatomy of the thyroid gland.

Thyroid anatomy

The thyroid gland is located beside the trachea, just below the larynx. It has two lobes, which are flat and oval, one on each side of the trachea, joined by an isthmus across the front of the trachea. The thyroid isthmus lies about halfway between the thyroid cartilage (the Adam's apple) and the sternal notch. The lobes are enclosed with two connective tissue capsules. In between these layers, the parathyroid glands are found. There are usually four parathyroid glands, found on the posterior surface of the thyroid gland. The recurrent laryngeal nerves are also found posteriorly between the thyroid and the trachea. Laterally, from anterior to posterior, the internal jugular vein, the vagus nerve and the common carotid artery are important relations (Fig. 7.1). The thyroid gland is not usually visible. When the thyroid gland increases in size it forms a characteristic swelling in the neck, called a 'goitre'.

What is a goitre?

This term refers to a swelling in the neck, caused by an enlarged thyroid (Fig. 7.2). The normal human thyroid gland is neither visible nor palpable. A thyroid has usually doubled in size in order to be palpable. To be visible, a thyroid has usually increased three-fold in size. Although the presence of a goitre is an indication of likely thyroid disease, it does not tell you anything about the underlying cause (Fig. 7.3). The thyroid is usually considered to weigh between 10 and 20 g; however, thyroid size varies hugely between individuals and between different geographical regions. In Iceland, the typical thyroid size is small because the population generally eats a diet rich in iodine. In other regions, normal thyroid size may be four to five times larger. Worldwide, the commonest cause of goitre is iodine deficiency.

So, the presence of a goitre indicates that the thyroid has grown abnormally large and suggests that investigation of thyroid function would be appropriate. The growth may be a result of low thyroid hormone secretion, resulting in high thyroid stimulating hormone (TSH) levels, which then stimulate thyroid growth (see below), or it may reflect an autonomous growth with excess thyroid hormone secretion (Fig. 7.3). A relatively common cause of an enlarged thyroid is the presence of auto-antibodies that act on the thyroid to stimulate growth and hormone secretion (Graves' disease).

Interesting fact

Some areas, such as Derbyshire, have low naturally occurring levels of iodine in the water supply. Goitre was formerly endemic in these areas, as drinking water was the major source of dietary iodine and goitre is still sometimes referred to as 'Derbyshire neck'. In the UK now, iodine deficiency goitre is very rare (see below).

Blood supply

The thyroid gland has a rich blood supply from the external carotid and subclavian arteries via the superior and inferior thyroid arteries (Fig. 7.1). The rate of blood flow through the gland is controlled by both sympathetic and

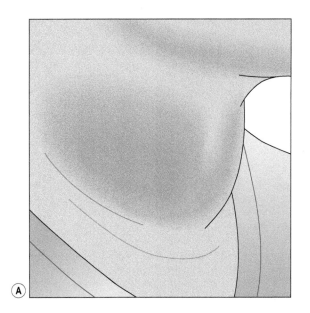

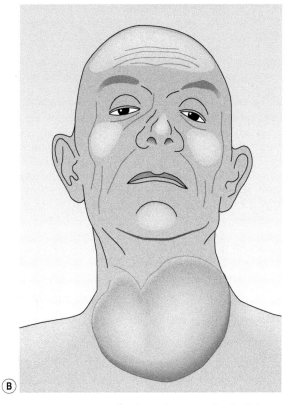

Figure 7.2 The appearance of goitre varies tremendously. Goitre can be a relatively small swelling around the neck, looking somewhat like a roll of fat (A) or much larger and more obviously nodular (B).

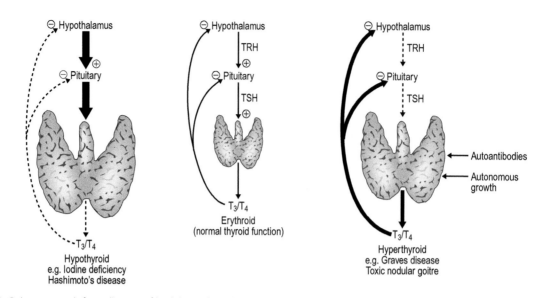

Figure 7.3 Goitre can result from diseases of both hyperthyroidism and hypothyroidism. In hyperthyroidism the stimulation is either autonomous or from antibodies, leading to thyroid growth and increased hormone output. In these cases TSH levels are extremely low. In hypothyroidism there is very low output of thyroid hormones so TSH levels are high, causing growth of the thyroid gland.

parasympathetic nerves. The normal rate of blood flow through the thyroid is around twice that of the kidney (at 3 mL/min/g or 30–60 mL/min through the gland), but in disorders involving growth of the thyroid tissue, such as diffuse toxic goitre, may reach 1 L/min in total. This can be detected with a stethoscope: there is an audible bruit over the gland.

Structure of the thyroid

The thyroid gland is made up of a large number of individual functional units called thyroid follicles. Each follicle consists of a single layer of follicular cells surrounding a pool of colloid, giving it an unmistakable appearance histologically (Fig. 7.4). On histological examination, when the section is stained with haematoxylin and eosin (H&E), the colloid appears pink and relatively homogeneous. The amount of colloid present varies according to the physiological status of the individual; there is more colloid present when the gland is inactive and almost none when the individual is iodine deficient. Among the follicular cells, are scattered C cells, which secrete calcitonin. These are larger than the follicular cells.

Synthesis of thyroid hormones

The thyroid gland makes active thyroid hormones by adding iodide residues to the amino acid tyrosine. Iodide is actively taken up into the follicular cells of the thyroid by a sodium/iodide symporter, which uses the sodium ion concentration gradient to enable the cells to take up iodide against a concentration gradient. This is a highly

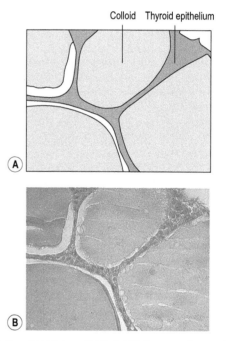

Figure 7.4 Thyroid histology. (A) Colloid is the smooth material stored in the space between cells. (B) This histological section of a thyroid gland shows thyroid follicles, with C cells showing as darkly staining cells in the parafollicular space. These are the calcitonin secreting cells (from Chew S L, Leslie D. 2006. Clinical endocrinology and diabetes: an illustrated colour text. Churchill Livingstone, Edinburgh, with permission.)

efficient process and up to 90% of dietary iodide can be taken up by the thyroid gland.

The follicular cells also synthesize a large protein, rich in tyrosine residues, called thyroglobulin which is secreted into a pool of colloid, which is surrounded by

Weight loss: 2

Case note: Why knowledge of anatomy is essential in his management

The fact that a neck mass is of thyroid origin can be shown by clinical examination and a knowledge of the anatomy and relations of the thyroid. The thyroid gland is wrapped in a layer of tissue called the pre-tracheal fascia, which is inserted into the trachea (Fig. 7.1). Thus, thyroid masses grow around the trachea and move with the trachea when the patient is asked to swallow. The trachea may become narrowed and even occluded by a thyroid mass, a potential medical and surgical emergency. The surgical anatomy of the thyroid gland is important in operations to remove the thyroid and in counselling patients about the risks of such procedures. The surgeon may have to contend with retrosternal extension, recurrent laryngeal nerve and parathyroid injury. The trachea often descends behind the sternum in older patients owing to a kyphosis of the neck; this is easily appreciated if the cricoid cartilage is found to be at the sternal notch.

Mr Smith's chest radiograph (Fig. 7.5) confirms that the thyroid is exerting pressure on the trachea and indicates a role for surgical removal once the overactive thyroid state has been fully controlled by medication.

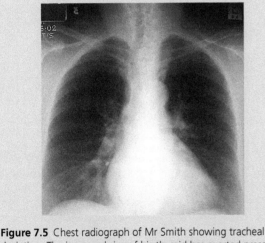

Figure 7.5 Chest radiograph of Mr Smith showing tracheal deviation. The increased size of his thyroid has exerted pressure on the trachea, causing it to be shifted to one side (from Chew S L, Leslie D. 2006. Clinical endocrinology and diabetes: an illustrated colour text. Churchill Livingstone, Edinburgh, with permission).

These iodinated tyrosine residues combine in pairs to form either tri-iodothyronine (T3) or tetra-iodothyronine (T4) (Figs 7.6, 7.7). When iodine is in short supply, however, it is common for the reaction to favour the formation of mono-iodotyrosine. So when there is a shortage of iodine, thyroid hormone synthesis favours T3 production over T4. These two hormones are the thyroid hormones. This iodinated colloid acts as a reserve of thyroid hormone for the body. Normally, the thyroid contains 5–6 weeks' supply of hormone. When the follicular cells are stimulated to produce thyroid hormones, droplets of the colloid are taken up by endocytosis into the cell, to form vesicles. These vesicles fuse with lysosomes, which contain enzymes that cut the thyroglobulin to release the pairs of iodinated tyrosine residues. While the iodothyronines are released into the blood, the remainder of the thyroglobulin is recycled in the follicular cell and used to make further colloid.

Iodine

Iodine is a monovalent anion, belonging to the same chemical group as chlorine: the halogens. It is a trace element in the diet and is essential for normal thyroid function. The UK Department of Health recommends a daily intake of 140 μg for most people and the World Health Organization suggests that pregnant and lactating women need 200 μg/day. In the diet, sea fish, shellfish and sea salt are particularly rich in iodine, reflecting the high iodine content of sea water. More surprisingly, perhaps, cow's milk is also a good source of iodine. Maybe this is not so surprising to people who are aware that iodine is used as a cattlefeed supplement and as a sterilizing agent applied to cow's teats in milking parlours. Iodine is also present in a wide range of multivitamin and mineral supplements. Dietary iodine deficiency is a serious public health problem (see below) and so, in the USA and many other countries, iodine is added as a supplement to table salt.

Interesting fact

While daily microgram quantities of iodide are essential for the thyroid to work properly, taking an excess of iodide (0.5 to 1.5 mg/day) paradoxically suppresses thyroid function and causes hypothyroidism. This is only a short-term effect however, and in the longer term the thyroid gland adapts to the increased supply of iodide and the person normally returns to the euthyroid state.

Thyroxine and T3: the thyroid hormones in blood

The active thyroid hormone is T3, but thyroxine can be converted to T3 in many tissues of the body, by a process called 'peripheral deiodination'. The thyroid gland

follicular cells. The iodide is also secreted into the lumen of the follicle by the action of a sodium-independent iodide transporter, called 'pendrin'. On the luminal (next to the colloid) surface of these cells, there is an enzyme, called thyroperoxidase, which catalyses the reaction between tyrosine residues in the thyroglobulin and the iodide, forming mono-iodotyrosine and di-iodotyrosine.

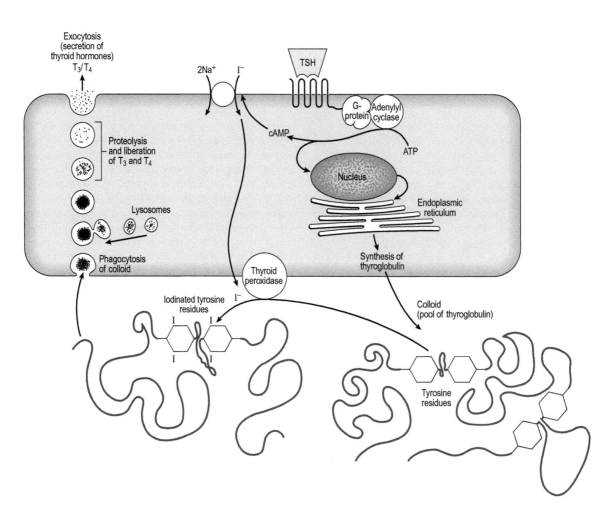

Figure 7.6 Synthesis of thyroid hormones. Iodine is actively concentrated by thyroid cells. An enzyme called thyroperoxidase catalyses the addition of iodine to the tyrosine residues in thyroglobulin, a large protein, rich in tyrosine residues, which is synthesized in thyroid cells. The iodinated thyroglobulin is stored in the thyroid in the form of 'colloid'. In response to TSH stimulation, portions of the colloid are taken back into the thyroid cell by phagocytosis and pairs of iodinated tyrosine residues (thyroxine) are released into the circulation. Anti-thyroid drugs, such as carbimazole, act by inhibiting thyroperoxidase activity. AC, adenylyl cyclase; cAMP, cyclic adenosine monophosphate.

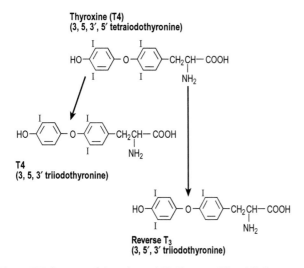

Figure 7.7 Structure of thyroxine and T3. These small lipophilic hormones act by binding to intracellular receptors. Thyroxine (T4) is converted to T3 or reverse T3 by de-iodination in peripheral tissues. Reverse T3 is inactive.

and the mechanism of peripheral de-iodination can also produce an inactive form of T3, called 'reverse T3' (Fig. 7.7). The thyroid hormones are poorly soluble in blood plasma and must therefore circulate in blood attached to a binding protein. In fact, 99.9% of thyroid hormone in blood is protein-bound. There are two plasma binding proteins for thyroid hormones. Thyroxine binding globulin (TBG) is the most important of these, binding approximately 70% of circulating thyroid hormones. The other is called transthyretin and binds only around 10% of thyroid hormones, less than the 15–20% that is loosely bound to serum albumin. Thyroxine binding globulin circulates in far lower concentrations than either transthyretin or albumin but it has a much higher affinity for thyroid hormones than the other proteins. It also has a long half-life of around 5 days compared with 2 days for transthyretin. Like other binding globulins, TBG is produced by the liver and is actively regulated, principally by oestrogens. This means that levels of TBG increase in pregnancy and in women taking the combined oral

Case 7.1 Weight loss: 3

Case note: Investigations

Mr Smith's doctor requested a thyroid function test, estimation of sex hormone binding globulin (SHBG) level, thyroid autoantibodies, and an ECG.

The following test results were obtained:

Free T4	28 pmol/L (normal, 9–25 pmol/L)
TSH	0.01 mU/L (normal, 0.4–4 mU/L)
Total T3	<10.8 nmol/L (normal, 1.2–2.2 nmol/L)
SHBG	135 nmol/L (normal male, 25–55 nmol/L)

Thyroid microsome autoantibodies   Negative

ECG   Atrial fibrillation, rate 140 b.p.m.

Interpretation of thyroid function test results

Mr Smith has abnormally high serum thyroxine (T4) and tri-iodothyronine (T3) levels. The normal thyroid produces mostly (80%) T4, and this is converted by loss of one iodine molecule (called de-iodination) to the active T3 by the tissues. The production of T4 is normally under the control of the pituitary hormone TSH. However, in Mr Smith's case, the thyroid nodules are autonomously making large amounts of T3 and some T4. The TSH is therefore inhibited by negative feedback effects of the thyroid hormones.

The thyroid hormones are stimulating the liver to produce SHBG, which is a marker of thyroid state and which binds and inactivates testosterone. The reduction in testosterone action allows an increased effect of oestrogen on breast tissue, causing hyperplasia. The latter fact explains the swollen breast tissue (called gynaecomastia).

An alternative diagnosis may have been auto-immune thyroid disease, in which thyroid autoantibodies are usually present. Thus, the negative thyroid autoantibodies result supports a diagnosis of toxic nodular goitre as opposed to Graves' disease.

The ECG confirms atrial fibrillation, which is a dangerous cardiac complication of thyrotoxicosis. Atrial fibrillation is a classical complication and carries a risk of stroke. Clots can form in the fibrillating atria and may move into the arterial system (a process called embolization).

contraceptive pill, but thyroid hormone secretion also increases so these women remain euthyroid. TBG levels are also raised in people taking methadone or heroin, and major tranquilizers, and decreased in people taking glucocorticoids or androgen therapy.

Thyroxine has an unusually long plasma half-life for a hormone, of around 6–7 days, while T3 has a shorter half-life of around 10 hours. The long half-life of thyroxine means that it does not have a significant diurnal rhythm and also that any drug treatment to reduce thyroid hormone secretion takes at least a week to have any significant effect on plasma hormone levels.

Control of thyroid function

The thyroid gland is regulated by a peptide hormone secreted from the anterior pituitary, quite sensibly called thyroid stimulating hormone (TSH). The control of thyroid hormone secretion is shown in Figure 7.8. This is a classical hypothalamic–pituitary axis, with thyroid hormones exerting negative feedback control of the axis. There is also inhibitory input from other hormones, including somatostatin and glucocorticoids. Examples of stimuli that increase activity of the hypothalamo–pituitary–thyroid axis include cold exposure, exercise and pregnancy. Thyroid stimulating hormone acts on specific receptors on the apical surface of the thyroid follicular cell (Fig. 7.6). The TSH receptor is a classical seven-transmembrane domain, G-protein coupled receptor

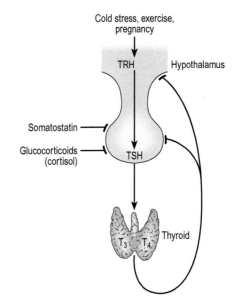

Figure 7.8 The hypothalamo–pituitary–thyroid axis.

linked to adenylyl cyclase. Activation of the receptor causes an increase in cAMP, which then brings about a range of intracellular responses to TSH stimulation over different time periods. The most immediate effect of TSH is to increase cellular uptake and processing of the colloid, to bring about the release of thyroid hormones. There is also an increase in iodide uptake and in synthesis

Case note: Establishing the diagnosis

Mr Smith is suffering from the effects of an excess of thyroid hormone (thyrotoxicosis), caused by a toxic nodular goitre. A goitre is an enlarged thyroid gland (see above). Most people over 40 years have small thyroid nodules detectable by high-resolution ultrasonography. Some of these nodules, in a minority of patients, will grow sufficiently to be seen or felt. Thyroid nodules may grow beyond normal control mechanisms and become autonomous. Autonomy means that the nodules produce thyroid hormones independently of control by the pituitary gland. Thus, the TSH level may fall while the nodule continues to produce thyroid hormones. Autonomous thyroid hormone production from the nodule then insidiously worsens until finally an excess of circulating thyroid hormones produces symptoms of thyrotoxicosis. Such thyroid glands are called 'toxic' for this reason.

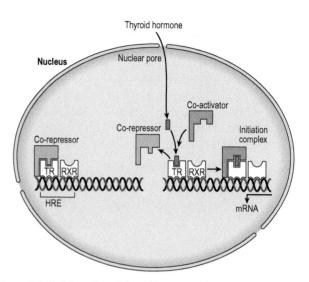

Figure 7.9 Cellular action of thyroid hormones. The thyroid hormone receptors (TR) are located in the nucleus of the target cell. They form dimers, either between two thyroid hormone receptors (homodimers) or with the retinoic acid receptor (RXR: heterodimers). In the absence of thyroid hormone they bind to a hormone response element in DNA and attract co-repressors which block gene transcription, but in the presence of thyroid hormone the co-repressors are replaced by co-activators, forming an initiation complex which allows gene transcription to proceed.

of thyroglobulin. In the longer term, TSH stimulates thyroid growth with both hyperplasia (increased size) and hypertrophy (increased number) of follicular cells. When there is excess TSH this leads to the development of a goitre (see above).

Cellular action of thyroid hormones

In the tissues, thyroid hormone diffuses across the plasma membrane into the cell and binds to specific receptors in the nucleus. There is a family of thyroid hormone receptors, which are encoded by two TR genes, alpha and beta. Alternative splicing of the gene products means that there are four distinct thyroid hormone receptors, with different tissue distributions and binding characteristics. These are TR alpha 1 and 2 and TR beta 1 and 2. TR alpha 2 is different from the other receptors because it does not bind T3 at all. The other receptors have a higher affinity for T3 than for T4. The TR beta 2 receptor is only found in the brain but the other receptors are found throughout the body. Unusually for nuclear receptors, the thyroid hormone receptors bind to the hormone response element on DNA even in the absence of thyroid hormones. The unoccupied receptors appear to have a role in repressing gene transcription, which is reversed when the hormone binds, allowing transcription to take place (Fig. 7.9). A key molecular target of thyroid hormone action is increased transcription of the genes encoding mitochondrial uncoupling proteins.

Effects of thyroid hormones

Thyroid hormones (Table 7.1) have a range of subtle effects in the body. Although the direct effects of these

Table 7.1   Actions of thyroid hormones

Cardiovascular effects:
  Increased cardiac output
  Increased heart rate and stroke volume
  Decreased systemic vascular resistance
  Increased systolic pressure

Metabolic effects:
  Increased basal metabolic rate
  Increased oxygen consumption
  Increased thermogenesis (increased expression of mitochondrial uncoupling proteins)
  Increased protein turnover (as a result of enhancing the actions of growth hormone, glucocorticoids, adrenaline, noradrenaline and glucagon)

Neurological effects
  Enhances
    Wakefulness
    Memory
    Alertness
    Reflexes
  Essential for maintenance of normal emotional tone

Growth and development
  Essential for normal fetal neural development
  Essential for normal bone growth after birth
  Required for normal tooth development

Reproduction
  Has a permissive role in both male and female reproduction: essential for normal reproductive function

hormones on particular tissues or cells may be subtle, both thyroid hormone insufficiency and excess result in significant disease. Like glucocorticoids, thyroid hormones do not have a single specific target tissue, but their receptors are found in most cells and tissues of the body. Although it is possible to state that cells need thyroid hormones to maintain their appropriate function, it has been difficult to identify their physiological effects.

Metabolic and respiratory effects

One of the main actions of thyroid hormones is to produce an increase in basal metabolic rate and an increase in the oxygen consumption and heat production of cells. Thyroid hormones achieve this by increasing expression of the genes which encode mitochondrial uncoupling proteins. Alongside this effect, thyroid hormones increase the resting respiratory rate and cause an increase in erythrocyte numbers by stimulating renal erythropoietin production. These effects work together over a time period of weeks to maintain blood oxygen levels when demand for oxygen is increased. Thyroid hormones also increase sweating, probably in response to the increased thermogenesis.

Cardiovascular effects

Thyroid hormones increase cardiac output both directly and indirectly (as a result of increased oxygen utilization and CO_2 production in the body). The direct cardiovascular effects of thyroid hormones include decreased peripheral resistance and increased stroke volume. Thyroid hormones act to alter responsiveness of cells to other hormones, especially to catecholamines and together they have a synergistic effect on heart rate.

Developmental effects

During fetal development and early childhood, thyroid hormones have an important role in both neural and skeletal development. Up to 11 weeks of fetal life, the developing fetus depends on the small amount of thyroxine that passes across the placenta from the maternal circulation. During the second trimester of pregnancy the fetal thyroid becomes active. Although there is a significant increase in circulating maternal thyroid hormones (see Ch. 9), this is accompanied by an increase in plasma binding globulin, so the concentration of free thyroxine is unchanged.

Other effects of thyroid hormones

At least partly by enhancing responsiveness to catecholamines, thyroid hormones affect the central nervous system. They are important in maintaining normal mood, memory formation and attention as well as in peripheral

---

Case 7.1 Weight loss: 5

Case note: Explanation of symptoms

Mr Smith's symptoms are due to an excess of thyroid hormones (thyrotoxicosis):

- Increased metabolic rate causes sweating, heat intolerance and weight loss despite good appetite
- Effects on skeletal muscle may cause proximal myopathy
- Effects on cardiac smooth muscle may cause atrial fibrillation (causing palpitations)
- Effects on brain cause agitation and labile mood
- Effects on β-adrenoceptors cause increased heart rate and peripheral tremor.

---

neural reflexes. Thyroid hormones have a role in maintaining healthy bones, skin, teeth and reproductive system. They are required for normal functioning of much of the endocrine system, have a role in regulating growth hormone secretion and in levels of expression of CYP19, the aromatase enzyme which converts androgens to oestrogens. It is difficult to overstate the importance of a properly functioning thyroid gland.

Disorders of thyroid hormone secretion

As we have seen, thyroid hormones have significant effects on virtually every system of the body. They affect metabolism, the cardiovascular system, the nervous system, bone, mood, the endocrine system and pretty much everything else. It is therefore not surprising that the effects of thyroid hormone excess or insufficiency are global and severe.

Disorders of the thyroid: hyperthyroidism

The diagnosis of an 'overactive thyroid' is relatively common. It has been estimated that up to 5% of British women have hyperthyroidism at some time in their lives, with half of these women having thyroid stimulating antibodies in their blood. Thyroid disorders are much less common in men. Hyperthyroidism results in a clinical condition called thyrotoxicosis, in which the levels of circulating thyroid hormones are so high that they cause symptoms (Fig 7.10).

The two commonest causes of thyrotoxicosis are toxic nodular goitre and Graves' disease. In both of these diseases, thyroid function is increased in the absence of stimulation from the pituitary. In toxic nodular disease there is an autonomous nodule in the thyroid gland that slowly increases thyroid hormone production. Graves' disease is an autoimmune condition in which auto-antibodies stimulate the TSH receptor. These antibodies were first recognized to be the cause of Graves' disease in the late 1950s although the clinical condition of

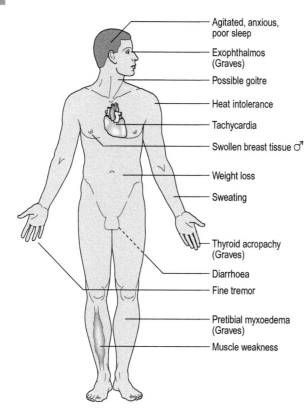

Agitated, anxious, poor sleep
Exophthalmos (Graves)
Possible goitre
Heat intolerance
Tachycardia
Swollen breast tissue ♂
Weight loss
Sweating
Thyroid acropachy (Graves)
Diarrhoea
Fine tremor
Pretibial myxoedema (Graves)
Muscle weakness

Figure 7.10 Signs and symptoms of hyperthyroidism (thyrotoxicosis).

Graves' disease itself was described in 1835. The autoantibodies take over control of the thyroid from TSH and so the usual negative feedback control does not work to limit thyroid hormone secretion. Graves' disease is part of a spectrum of organ-specific autoimmune disease, including conditions such as pernicious anaemia. Both toxic nodular goitre and Graves' disease cause the symptoms of excess thyroid hormone secretion (see below), but additional signs and symptoms are seen in Graves' disease. In particular, effects on the eye are seen, upper lid retraction and exophthalmos being most noticeable (Fig. 7.11). Graves' disease is also associated with vitiligo (patchy skin depigmentation), myxoedema (thickening of the skin on the lower legs) and finger clubbing.

Interesting fact

Thyroxine is available over the internet as an 'aid to weight loss'. A quick glance at the effects of excess thyroid hormones should be enough to convince you of the foolishness of this course of action. Thyroxine supplements should be taken only on the advice of a qualified doctor.

Effects of excess thyroid hormone secretion: thyrotoxicosis

Thyroid hormones have effects on most tissues of the body, and the effects of excess thyroxine are exaggerations of the

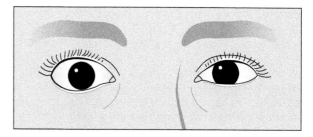

Figure 7.11 Graves' exophthalmia (proptosis). In this case, only one eye is affected. A combination of fat deposition behind the eyes and retraction of the eyelids causes this effect, which is characteristic of Graves' disease and is probably an effect of the antibodies rather than the increased levels of thyroid hormones.

normal physiological actions (Fig. 7.10). The increased basal metabolic rate makes the person feel hot and sweaty. This is often noticed by the individual as heat intolerance, feeling hot even in cool temperatures. As glycolysis increases, there is increased demand for glucose, so both weight loss and increased appetite are often seen together. The general catabolic state leads to a loss of muscle mass, which leads to muscle weakness. This is most noticeable in the large muscles around the hip and shoulder.

Thyroid hormones alter the actions of other hormones, especially the catecholamines, so tachycardia (increased heart rate) is seen. The tachycardia is a very serious problem which may be associated with atrial fibrillation, heart failure and death. Thyrotoxicosis is therefore a significant illness and should be treated promptly. The enhanced adrenergic effect also causes a peripheral tremor—typically a fine tremor of the hands. There are effects on mood, and excess thyroid hormones can cause elation, restlessness, anxiety or irritability. Excess thyroid hormones can also cause diarrhoea, by directly stimulating gut motility, and menstrual irregularities. The menstrual irregularities arise from a combination of weight loss and direct effects of the thyroid hormones on hypothalamic and pituitary hormones.

Treatment of thyrotoxicosis

The aim of treatment of thyrotoxicosis is to reduce the rate of secretion of thyroid hormones and to bring circulating levels of thyroid hormones and TSH within the normal range. There are several different ways in which this can be achieved. The first-line treatment is therapy with anti-thyroid drugs, such as carbimazole (methimazole). In some cases, this is used as a long-term treatment and in others it is used to reduce the size of a goitre prior to surgical treatment of the hyperthyroidism. Anti-thyroid drugs act by inhibiting the synthesis of thyroid hormones. Carbimazole (methimazole) is the most commonly used anti-thyroid drug in the UK. It acts by inhibiting the iodination of tyrosine residues on thyroglobulin. It is thought to do this by competing with tyrosine for binding to the thyroperoxidase enzyme. Propylthiouracil, another anti-thyroid drug has a similar mechanism of action in the thyroid, but it additionally inhibits the conversion of T4 to T3 in peripheral tissues and so its effects may be seen more rapidly. Typically the effects of anti-thyroid drugs take 4–6 weeks to become apparent. This is due to both the long half-life of thyroxine in the circulation, and the large reserve of iodinated thyroglobulin stored in the thyroid gland.

An alternative treatment for thyrotoxicosis is to use radioactively labelled iodine. The thyroid gland is the only organ in the body to trap iodine with great efficiency and thus radioiodine will localize nearly exclusively to the thyroid and will painlessly and safely destroy the thyroid tissue over a period of several weeks to months. With all antithyroid treatments, it is easy to go too far and get hypothyroidism so very often a 'blocking-replacement' treatment is used where the aim is to completely block endogenous thyroid hormone secretion and to give a replacement dose of thyroxine. Beta blockers such as propranolol are often used for immediate relief of the symptoms caused by enhanced adrenergic activity such as tremor and arrhythmias.

Case 7.1 — Weight loss: 6

Case note: Treatment

There are several aims in treating Mr Smith:

1. Control of thyroid hormone levels.
2. Treatment of atrial fibrillation and its complications.
3. Long-term treatment of the nodular goitre.

Mr Smith was started on the anti-thyroid drug, carbimazole. However, it usually takes several weeks for the drug to be fully effective and the tissue effects of thyrotoxicosis may take weeks to resolve after the introduction of anti-thyroid drugs. Thus, the β-adrenoceptor blocking drug, propranolol, was also started. High thyroid hormone levels act together with catecholamines to stimulate the heart and tissues. Blocking the β-adrenoceptor may improve some symptoms in many patients.

The treatment of Mr Smith's atrial fibrillation is essential, as there is a risk of clot formation in the heart with embolization to the brain and other parts of the vascular tree. Mr Smith was therefore given warfarin (an anticoagulant) to reduce the risk of clots.

Nodular goitres may be treated by surgery or radioactive iodine. A treatment plan for Mr Smith was made which included the use of radioactive iodine several weeks after he had been rendered clinically and biochemically euthyroid by drug treatment.

Causes of thyroid hyposecretion

Globally, hypothyroidism is most commonly caused by dietary iodine deficiency, although this is not usually seen in Western societies. There are also autoimmune causes, and hypothyroidism may result from insufficient pituitary secretion of TSH, although this is uncommon.

Iodine deficiency hypothyroidism

The thyroid gland has an absolute requirement for a supply of iodine in the diet. The World Health Organization recently reported that 30% of the world's population is at risk of iodine deficiency disorders. Children born to severely iodine-deficient mothers have a condition of severe mental retardation termed cretinism, which is the result of a lack of thyroid hormones. At the start of the 21st century, 750 million people were reported to suffer from iodine deficiency goitre. Some 43 million people have brain damage resulting from a deficiency of iodine and therefore of thyroid hormones. This is the commonest preventable cause of brain damage in the world today.

Autoimmune thyroid disease

There are several autoimmune disorders such as Hashimoto's thyroiditis, which cause impaired thyroid hormone secretion. These disorders are caused by autoantibodies directed against thyroglobulin or thyroid peroxidase. These antibodies cause progressive destruction of the thyroid gland which is often associated with local inflammation and pain. Like Graves' disease, autoimmune thyroiditis is 10–20 times more common in women than in men and has a peak occurrence between the ages of 45 and 65.

Effects of thyroid hormone insufficiency: myxoedema

The symptoms of hypothyroidism in adults develop only slowly, over a long period of time. Symptoms are often of general tiredness and lethargy. There may be weight gain despite poor appetite. Hypothyroidism causes depression in about 50% of cases, as well as cognitive impairment, a general sluggishness of intellectual process. There is reduced cardiac output and the pulse rate is slow (Fig. 7.12).

Congenital hypothyroidism

In children, hypothyroidism is very serious and can result in severe brain damage. Congenital hypothyroidism occurs in about 1 in 4000 children born in the UK. This relatively high incidence, combined with the seriousness of the condition and its simple treatment once detected, mean that a national screening programme has been introduced in the UK. All babies born in the UK have a heel-prick blood test when they are about 7 days old. The blood spot is tested for thyroid hormones and thyroxine treatment is started if there is evidence of hypothyroidism. There is good evidence that thyroid hormone replacement prevents the consequences of hypothyroidism in these children, although it does not correct any damage that occurred before birth.

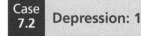

Case 7.2   Depression: 1

Case history

Ms Cooper, a 54-year-old bank executive, was referred to the psychiatry outpatients for assessment of her depression, which was resistant to treatment. She had felt increasingly depressed over the past 6 months and had presented to her GP 6 weeks earlier, whereupon treatment with an antidepressant had been started. This had had no effect on her mood and other symptoms, to the point where Ms Cooper was becoming suicidal. She described low mood, lack of energy and lack of enjoyment – the three core features of depression.

Ms Cooper had been unable to work for the past month and had considerable difficulty concentrating. She was very pessimistic about the future and felt guilty that she was unable to 'snap out of it'. Her appetite was decreased, but she had not lost weight, despite eating much less than usual. She reported increased sleep at night and daytime sleepiness.

Ms Cooper had no history of psychiatric disorders or other significant illness. There was no family history of depression or other psychiatric disorder, but Ms Cooper's mother had a history of hypothyroidism.

On direct questioning, Ms Cooper described how she had been feeling tired and run down for over a year and that she had become intolerant of cold, wearing thick winter clothing on a warm August day. Normally she was very energetic, with a busy lifestyle, and was particularly distressed that she had had to gradually give up more and more of her activities due to her tiredness and lack of concentration.

A thyroid function test was requested. The results were:

Free T4   6.7 pmol/L (normal, 9–25 pmol/L)

TSH   112 mU/L (normal, 0.4–4 mU/L)

Ms Cooper was started on 50 μg thyroxine/day and was stabilized on 125 μg/day.

Within 3 weeks of starting thyroxine treatment her mood had lifted, tiredness decreased, she felt less sleepy and her appetite had increased. Some 3 weeks later she had made a full recovery, returned to work and started some other activities. At this point, the antidepressant medication was stopped.

This case raises the question: Why was a thyroid function test requested rather than alternative forms of antidepressant treatment?

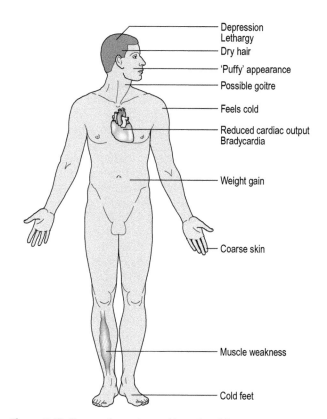

Figure 7.12 Signs and symptoms of hypothyroidism.

Treatment of hypothyroidism

Thyroxine replacement is given to treat hypothyroidism. It is active orally and so can be taken in tablet form. The long half-life of thyroxine in blood means that it can be taken once daily. The aim of treatment is to bring the patient into a 'euthyroid' state. This is best judged, in patients with an intact pituitary, by measuring plasma TSH levels. The aim of treatment is to keep the plasma thyroxine at a level where TSH is just suppressed below about 4 mU/L. This usually requires 'titration' of the dose of thyroxine (i.e. a process of trial and error).

Interesting fact

One of the simplest and most effective measures put in place to improve public health across the world has been the addition of iodine to table salt to prevent the mental retardation caused by thyroxine deficiency. Iodine and foods rich in iodine have long been known as a treatment for goitre—in Chinese medicine seaweed is used. Since the early 20th century, salt manufacturers have added iodine, usually in the form of potassium iodide, to table salt. Although the World Health Organization strongly supports iodization of salt, it is not a universally popular measure.

HORMONAL CONTROL OF REPRODUCTION PART I:
MALE REPRODUCTIVE SYSTEM

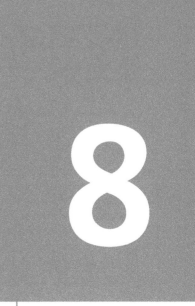

Chapter objectives

After studying this chapter you should be able to:

1. Describe the structure and function of the testes.

2. Explain the control of steroid hormone production by the testes.

3. Describe the hormonal regulation of spermatogenesis.

4. Understand the endocrine abnormalities that may affect men's sexual health.

5. Describe the uses of androgens as therapeutic drugs and substances of abuse.

Introduction

The male reproductive system has two functions. First is the production of the male gamete, called sperm, by a process called spermatogenesis. The second is the production of the male sex hormones, a class of steroid hormones called the androgens, which are necessary for spermatogenesis to occur and also maintain sexual potency and secondary sex characteristics. The testes, or testicles (Fig. 8.1), are the pair of male gonads (the singular is testis) and the principal androgen is testosterone. Testicular function is controlled by the hypothalamo–pituitary–testicular axis which regulates both androgen synthesis and spermatogenesis.

Where are the testes?

It may not come as a big surprise to learn that the testes are located outside the abdominal wall, in a sac called the scrotum (Fig. 8.1). During fetal life, the testes develop within the abdomen, and descend to the scrotum during the later stages of fetal development. The location of the testes is significant; spermatogenesis requires a temperature somewhat lower than normal body temperature and this is achieved by locating the testes in the scrotum. In an adult male, each testis is usually 20–25 mL in volume. In a small proportion of boys (approximately 3% of baby boys delivered at term, but 30% of pre-term boys) at least one testis has failed to descend fully into the scrotum, a condition known as cryptorchidism (meaning 'hidden testis'), which is treated surgically (Fig. 8.2). During fetal development, the testes descend from the abdominal cavity into the scrotum via a gap in the abdominal wall called the inguinal canal. The route of descent of the testes is shown in Figure 8.2. Failure of the inguinal canal to fully close can allow a loop of intestine to also pass through and become trapped. This results in a very common condition called an inguinal hernia.

Interesting fact

The fact that a relatively low temperature is required for spermatogenesis has led to the myth that taking a hot bath before sexual intercourse diminishes a man's fertility enough to act as a contraceptive. Given that the process of sperm maturation takes 70 days, it would need to be a very long hot bath!

Like many myths, this one has its basis in fact. Over the longer term, conservative measures like wearing looser clothing and avoiding hot baths can improve fertility in sub-fertile men.

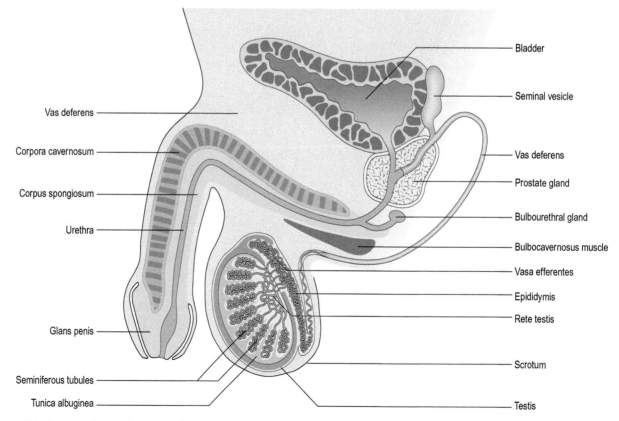

Figure 8.1 Structure of the male reproductive system.

What are the testes?

The testes are made up of two functional parts: the seminiferous tubules and Leydig cells (Fig. 8.3). The bulk of the testicular volume (approximately 90%) is made up of seminiferous tubules, which give the testis its lobular appearance. Each seminiferous tubule would be about 60 cm long if stretched out, but luckily is tightly coiled within the testis. The seminiferous tubules are the location of spermatogenesis. The second functional part of the testis, comprising the Leydig cells (or interstitial cells), lies between the seminiferous tubules (Fig. 8.4). The Leydig cells can function independently of the seminiferous tubules. However, the seminiferous tubules need functioning Leydig cells.

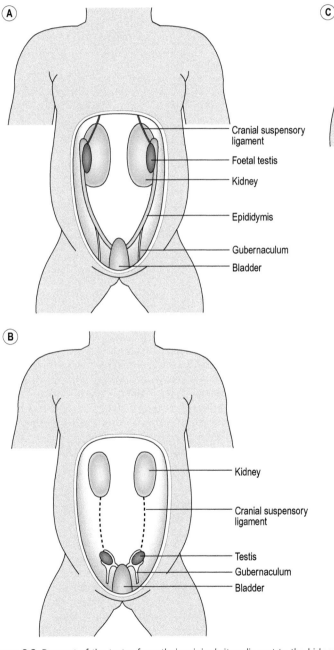

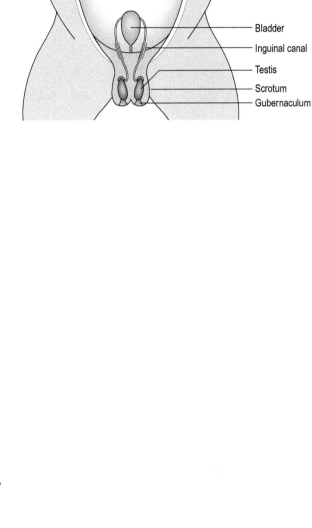

Figure 8.2 Descent of the testes from their original site adjacent to the kidney into the scrotum. This is a complex process and the testis can become 'stuck' at almost any point during its descent (A). The fetal testis is held next to the kidney by the cranial suspensory ligament. It is also attached to the gubernaculum testis, a jelly-like ligament that connects the testis and epididymis to the scrotum. The action of androgens causes this ligament to dissolve, and the action of growth factors causes the gubernaculum to contract. The combined effect is that the testis is drawn into the lower abdomen adjacent to the inguinal canal at around 12 weeks' gestation (B). Under the influence of androgens, the testis passes through the inguinal canal into the scrotum between 27 and 30 weeks' gestation (C).

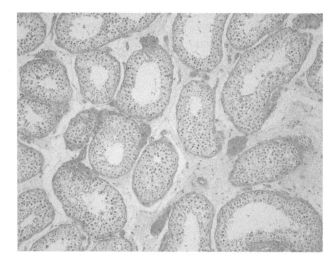

Figure 8.3 Histological appearance of the testis. (Courtesy of Dr Dan Berney.)

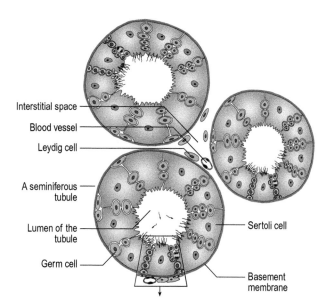

Interstitial space

Blood vessel

Leydig cell

A seminiferous tubule

Lumen of the tubule

Germ cell

Sertoli cell

Basement membrane

Figure 8.4 Structure of the testes showing the arrangement of seminiferous tubules and a section through a seminiferous tubule. The area in the box is shown in more detail in Figure 8.5.

The seminiferous tubules consist of two cell types: Sertoli cells and germ cells (Fig. 8.5). At puberty, there are around 600 million germ cells, called spermatogonia, per testis. The Sertoli cells provide both nutrition and hormonal support to allow the germ cells to develop into sperm, and functional Sertoli cells are required for spermatogenesis to occur. Each Sertoli cell is in contact with a number of germ cells. However, the relationship between the germ cells and Sertoli cells is not fully understood. The seminiferous tubules lead to the epididymis, where sperm maturation occurs. The epididymis is connected to the urethra by the vas deferens (Fig. 8.1).

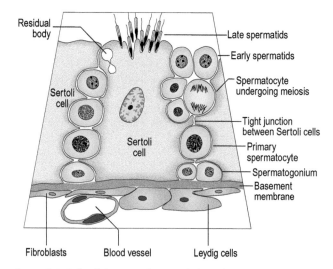

Residual body

Sertoli cell

Sertoli cell

Late spermatids

Early spermatids

Spermatocyte undergoing meiosis

Tight junction between Sertoli cells

Primary spermatocyte

Spermatogonium

Basement membrane

Fibroblasts   Blood vessel   Leydig cells

Figure 8.5 Cells of the seminiferous tubule and the process of spermatogenesis. The germ cells originate next to the basement membrane, between the Sertoli cells. As these germ cells, known as spermatogonia, develop, they migrate towards the lumen of the seminiferous tubule, passing between the Sertoli cells. The immature spermatids are released from the secondary spermatogonia into the lumen of the seminiferous tubule, leaving 'residual bodies' behind. The spermatids mature into spermatozoa as they pass along the tubules and through the epididymis.

There is a blood–testis barrier, formed by the very tight contact between adjacent Sertoli cells. This barrier has an important role in maintaining an internal environment within the testis that is different from the blood or extracellular fluid. The intra-testicular fluid contains a testosterone binding protein which has an important role in maintaining a high intra-testicular testosterone concentration. The blood–testis barrier also functions to prevent fragments of immature sperm from entering the bloodstream and triggering an immune response. Disruption of the blood–testis barrier has been proposed as the triggering event in the production of anti-sperm antibodies, resulting in sub-fertility. It is also thought that this barrier may protect sperm to some extent from blood-borne toxins.

Testicular blood and nerve supply

Blood supply to each testis is independent and originates mainly through the left or right testicular artery, which arise from the aorta. However, the testicular artery forms a network of connections with the internal iliac artery, which supplies the vas deferens, so that the blood supply to the testis effectively has two origins. Venous drainage is into the inferior vena cava on the right and the renal vein on the left. It is thought that the dual-origin blood supply may protect the testis from possible disruption. However, as the testis descends from the abdomen into the scrotum, it trails its blood vessels and nerves behind it. During the process of testicular descent, or at a later stage in life, the testis can twist, causing restriction of

Unexpected fracture: 1

Case history

John Smith, a 25-year-old man, came to the A&E department after a fall. He had tripped while crossing the road and had fallen awkwardly. The main impact was on the right side of the chest. After the fall he had severe chest pain over the site of the impact.

The past medical history was unremarkable. Mr Smith was taking no medications and did not smoke or drink alcohol. He lived with his wife and worked as a chef. The couple had been attempting to have a baby for 2 years, with no success.

The examination showed him to be tall with long arms and legs. There was swelling of breast tissue underlying the nipple on both sides. The doctor found the right lower ribs to be very tender and there was bruising over the skin. There was scanty body, pubic and axillary hair, and the testes were very small (<2 mL in volume; normal, ≥20 mL).

Chest radiography revealed several fractures in the right lower ribs. The doctor was concerned about the severity of the fractures despite the relatively trivial fall. The doctor was also concerned about the other findings on clinical examination.

the blood supply or impaired venous drainage, which is treated as a surgical emergency.

The nerve supply to the testis is from the sympathetic chain from the thoracic spine. The vas deferens receives a parasympathetic nerve supply from the pelvic chain. The sympathetic supply controls erection while the parasympathetic supply controls ejaculation. An intact nerve supply is therefore essential for normal sexual function.

Spermatogenesis

Spermatogenesis is the process by which the germ cells in the seminiferous tubules develop into mature sperm (Fig. 8.5). There are three distinct stages to this process: proliferation of the spermatogonia, reduction of the number of chromosomes (meiosis) and development of the mature sperm structure. The spermatogonia are not used up during this process: after the second division of each stem cell, three of the spermatogonia continue on the pathway of cell division that leads to the production of sperm, while the fourth remains as a stem cell and begins dividing again to produce more spermatogonia. A healthy man produces around 200 million sperm every day, from puberty to old age. This adds up to several trillion sperm over a lifetime. The whole process, from the start of spermatogonium differentiation to the formation of a mature sperm, takes 70 days, with a further 12–21 days required for transport of the sperm through the epididymis to the ejaculatory duct. Each spermatogonium gives rise to a total of 64 sperm. Each ejaculate contains approximately 200 million sperm, with the volume of the ejaculate (usually around 3 mL) made up of fluids from the seminal vesicles and prostate gland.

Interesting fact

Vasectomy is an irreversible form of contraception. A vasectomy is performed by cutting both of the vas deferens (Fig. 8.1) and tying the cut ends. This prevents sperm from entering the ejaculate. A man who has had a vasectomy is still able to maintain an erection and to produce ejaculate as normal, due to the intact endocrine functions of the testis, but as no sperm are able to get through the cut vas deferens he is effectively infertile. He still produces sperm but these are simply absorbed back into the body. One interesting effect of vasectomy is the appearance of antibodies against spermatozoa; this occurs in about half of all vasectomized men. It is not known why this occurs but it contributes to the problems associated with attempted reversal of the vasectomy procedure.

Androgen production

The Leydig cell produces androgens which, like all steroid hormones, are made from cholesterol (Fig. 8.6). A range of androgens is made in the body and, although most of these come from the testes, some are made in the adrenal cortex (see Ch. 6). The most potent and important of these androgens is testosterone, and by far the highest production of testosterone is in the testes. The testis is not a highly vascular tissue like the adrenal cortex, and the presence of the blood–testis barrier and a specific androgen binding protein in the interstitial fluid of the testis means that high concentrations of testosterone accumulate. These high local levels of testosterone in the testis are important for spermatogenesis.

Hormonal control of testicular function

Both spermatogenesis and androgen secretion are controlled by the hypothalamus and pituitary glands (Fig. 8.7). The hypothalamic hormone, gonadotropin releasing hormone (GnRH), is secreted in a pulsatile manner to stimulate luteinizing hormone (LH) and follicle stimulating hormone (FSH) secretion. This pulsatile pattern of secretion is important: if GnRH is given as a constant infusion it actually inhibits secretion of these hormones (see below).

Control of testosterone secretion (Leydig cell function)

LH acts on the Leydig cells to stimulate testosterone synthesis. It binds to specific G-protein coupled receptors, linked to adenylyl cyclase and so increases cAMP production. The actions of LH on the Leydig cell are very

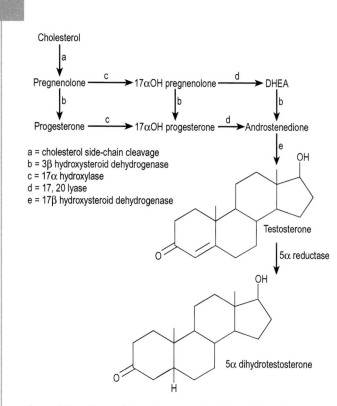

Figure 8.6 Pathway of testosterone synthesis in Leydig cells and of 5α-dihydrotestosterone in peripheral tissues. Cholesterol is the starting point for steroid biosynthesis in all steroid secreting tissues. The key shows all the enzyme activities involved in this biosynthetic pathway.

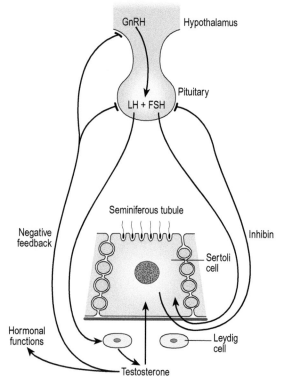

Figure 8.7 Hypothalamo–pituitary–testis axis. Gonadotropin releasing hormone (GnRH), released from the hypothalamus, stimulates the gonadotroph cells of the anterior pituitary to release luteinizing hormone (LH) and follicle stimulating hormone (FSH). LH acts on Leydig cells to stimulate testosterone production, which acts with FSH on Sertoli cells to stimulate spermatogenesis. Testosterone and inhibin, a peptide secreted by Sertoli cells, exert negative feedback control of this axis.

similar to the actions of ACTH on the adrenal cell (see Ch. 6), with the involvement of StAR protein transporting cholesterol to the inner mitochondrial membrane to initiate steroidogenesis (Fig. 8.8).

There is negative feedback inhibition of the hypothalamo–pituitary–testicular axis, with testosterone inhibiting LH secretion. In addition to the effects of testosterone on LH secretion, there are two peptide hormones secreted by the Sertoli cells that also have a role in regulating this axis: activin, which stimulates GnRH and FSH secretion, and inhibin, which inhibits FSH secretion.

In common with the hypothalamo–pituitary–adrenal axis, there is marked diurnal variation in the activity of the hypothalamo–pituitary–testicular axis. Plasma testosterone levels in normal men peak at around 0700 hours and decline during the day to reach a nadir of around 60% of peak levels by early evening. The clinical significance of this variation has only recently been recognized and it is now recommended that plasma testosterone is sampled in the morning as there can be a 25% decline in plasma testosterone between 1000 hours and 1600 hours.

Control of spermatogenesis (Sertoli cell function)

Testosterone secreted by the Leydig cells acts together with FSH on the Sertoli cells to stimulate spermatogenesis (Fig. 8.7). The process of spermatogenesis is

absolutely dependent on the presence of an appropriate level of testosterone within the testis. However, although FSH stimulates Sertoli cell spermatogenesis, a low level of this activity can occur in the absence of FSH. Like LH (Fig. 8.8), FSH binds to a G-protein-coupled receptor and stimulates adenylyl cyclase activity. However, a number of other pathways are also activated, including several kinase cascades. The action of testosterone on Sertoli cells appears to involve a membrane receptor coupled to the opening of ligand-gated ion channels, in addition to the more usual transcriptional effects expected of a steroid.

We have already seen that Sertoli cells also have an endocrine function, with the secretion of the regulatory peptides activin and inhibin. Inhibin may be used as a marker of Sertoli cell function as serum concentrations of this hormone are directly related to sperm count.

In addition to stimulating spermatogenesis, FSH also causes the Sertoli cells to produce an androgen binding protein (ABP). This protein binds testosterone and helps maintain a high concentration of testosterone within the testes; this is essential for spermatogenesis to occur.

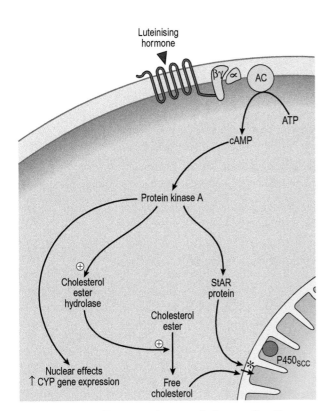

Figure 8.8 Effects of luteinizing hormone (LH) on Leydig cells. Binding of LH to its receptor activates (via a G-protein, Gs) adenylyl cyclase (AC), which causes an increase in intracellular cyclic adenosine monophosphate (cAMP), resulting in activation of cAMP-dependent kinase. This phosphorylates and activates cholesterol ester hydrolase, liberating free cholesterol from intracellular pools, and also causes an increase in steroidogenic acute regulatory (StAR) protein. StAR protein facilitates the transport of cholesterol from the outer to the inner mitochondrial membrane (shown by an asterisk), allowing cholesterol access to the first enzyme of steroidogenesis: cholesterol side-chain cleavage (P450scc). The rate of transfer of cholesterol from the outer to the inner mitochondrial membrane is what determines the rate of steroidogenesis—called the 'rate limiting step'.

Interesting fact

High concentrations of testosterone within the testes are required to support spermatogenesis, whereas only relatively low concentrations are needed to maintain potency (the ability to have and maintain an erection) and secondary sexual characteristics of men. This difference has been the basis for the development of a hormonal form of male contraceptive (see Ch. 10).

Transport of testosterone in blood

Testosterone is transported in blood bound to a carrier protein, called either testosterone binding globulin (TeBG) or, more commonly, sex hormone binding globulin (SHBG). In healthy men, only about 2% of the circulating testosterone is unbound, with 44% bound to SHBG and 54% bound to serum albumin. The protein-bound testosterone is protected from metabolism in the liver and provides an easily accessible pool of hormone, as the testosterone readily dissociates from its binding protein. Levels of SHBG in plasma are regulated by androgens, oestrogens and thyroid hormones. In healthy men, SHBG levels are fairly constant, but may need to be considered when steroid replacement therapy is used. Plasma testosterone concentrations are around 9–41 nmol/L in healthy men and 1–3 nmol/L in women. Plasma testosterone tends to decrease with age in men. Testosterone is metabolized in the liver, mostly to form androsterone and aetiocholanolone, which are excreted in urine.

Actions of testosterone

Testosterone has two main actions: the initiation of spermatogenesis and the development and maintenance of secondary sexual characteristics. In order to achieve the second group of actions, testosterone must be converted to 5α-dihydrotestosterone (DHT) (see Fig. 8.6). This conversion happens outside the testes, in peripheral tissues. Consequently, testosterone is sometimes described as a 'pre-hormone' or hormonal precursor, although this is not really correct as testosterone itself has a number of direct actions, including a range of metabolic effects as well as the maintenance of spermatogenesis. Furthermore, both testosterone and DHT act on the same receptor, the androgen receptor (AR). In general, when the actions of testosterone are described, the effects of DHT are included in the description.

Cellular actions of androgens

As steroids, testosterone and DHT act on an intracellular receptor, the androgen receptor, to alter the rate of transcription of certain genes and thus increase the production of certain proteins (Fig. 8.9). The androgen receptor is located in the cytoplasm of target cells, and in the absence of ligand it is associated with a chaperone protein called heat shock protein. When an androgen binds to the receptor the heat shock protein dissociates from the receptor, which then moves into the nucleus and forms a dimer with another androgen receptor. This dimer binds to an androgen response element on a gene promoter and also binds a number of co-activator proteins. Together, this complex is able to activate gene transcription. Given that both testosterone and DHT bind to the same receptor, it is not clear why the formation of DHT is necessary for some of the actions of testosterone. A defect in the gene encoding the androgen receptor can cause androgen insensitivity. The developmental consequences of this are considered in Chapter 10.

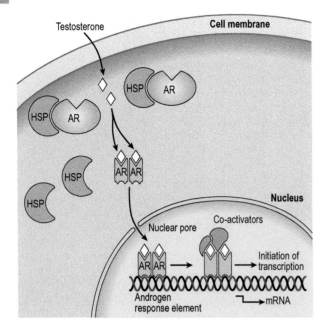

Figure 8.9 Cellular actions of androgens. Androgen receptors are intracellular and in the absence of testosterone they are bound to heat shock protein (HSP) and located in the cytoplasm. In the presence of androgen the HSP dissociates from the receptor allowing the hormone receptor complex to move into the nucleus where it dimerizes with another androgen receptor–hormone complex and binds to the androgen response element on a gene promoter. Various co-activators are attracted to the complex and gene transcription occurs.

Interesting fact

The androgen receptor (AR) is encoded by a gene located on the X-chromosome, so each male has just one copy of this gene, while paradoxically every female has two copies. This means that mutations of the AR gene are inherited as an X-linked recessive condition, known as androgen insensitivity syndrome (AIS), with carrier mothers having a 50% chance of passing the defective gene on to their sons. As with other X-linked recessive conditions, AIS affects almost exclusively men, although some carrier women may have a partial effect with sparse pubic and axillary hair. Affected men with complete AIS are genetically male (46XY) but phenotypically female (see also Ch. 10).

Physiological actions of androgens

The main physiological actions of testosterone and DHT are shown in Figure 8.10 and Table 8.1. In puberty, testosterone stimulates growth of long bones, causing an initial growth spurt, but then leads to fusing of the epiphyseal plates, resulting in cessation of long bone growth. Testosterone also causes laryngeal growth, which results in deepening of the voice at puberty; this is pronounced in boys, but much less so in girls. In boys at puberty, testosterone causes growth of the penis, scrotum, prostate, seminal vesicles, epididymis and vas deferens.

In an adult man, testosterone is essential for the maintenance of secondary sexual characteristics. It enhances

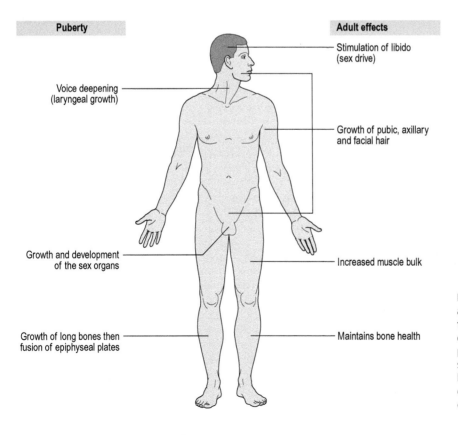

Figure 8.10 Actions of androgens. The actions specific to puberty are shown on the left and effects in adult men are shown on the right. The actions shown are mainly physiological effects on men. However, it should be noted that in women testosterone has an important role in stimulating libido, even though it circulates in only very low concentrations.

Table 8.1 Actions of androgens in men

Intrauterine:

 Development of male phenotype

 Development of penis, scrotum, prostate, etc.

 Testicular descent into scrotum

 Programming of male behaviour

At puberty:

 Development of male secondary sex characteristics

 Hypertrophy of larynx (deepening of voice)

 Development of seminal vesicles and prostate and initiation of sperm production

 Increased muscle mass

 Increased skin thickness and sebum formation

 Development of pubic and axillary hair

 Fusion of epiphyseal plates in long bone

In the adult man:

 Reproductive effects

  Maintenance of spermatogenesis

  Maintenance of secondary sex characteristics including beard growth

  Maintenance of libido (sex drive)

  Feedback inhibition of hypothalamic GnRH secretion

 Metabolic effects

  Lipid metabolism, increasing circulating VLDL and LDL, decreasing HDL

  Increased metabolic rate

  Increased red blood cell number

  Maintenance of muscle mass

  Maintenance of bone density

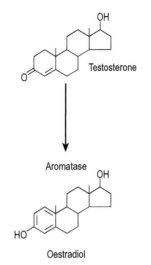

Figure 8.11 Conversion of testosterone to 17β-oestradiol by the actions of aromatase, an enzyme found in adipose tissues.

libido, is necessary for getting and maintaining an erection (potency), and stimulates the growth of facial, pubic and axillary hair. Testosterone is also necessary for bone health: testosterone deficiency causes osteoporosis. Testosterone is an anabolic androgenic steroid and has a range of metabolic effects, acting to increase lean body mass, to stimulate red blood cell production and to alter plasma lipid composition. It also causes growth of skeletal muscle, an effect that is exploited by some athletes and body-builders (see below).

Actions of oestrogens in men

It may seem surprising that many of the actions of testosterone are brought about, not by testosterone itself, but by an oestrogen. Androgens can be readily interconverted to oestrogens through the actions of an enzyme called aromatase (Fig. 8.11). This enzyme is encoded by a member of the *CYP* family of steroid hydroxylase genes, *CYP19*. This gene is expressed in adipose tissue, brain and testis. In oestrogen-dependent tissues or cells, the aromatase enzyme is co-located with the oestrogen receptor. Circulating levels of oestrogens are very low in healthy men, but circulating testosterone, converted locally by aromatase, may then have local oestrogenic actions.

Oestrogens are responsible for a wide range of actions in men. They act on the brain to affect sex drive and behaviour as well as mediating part of the negative feedback effects of testosterone on the hypothalamo–pituitary–testicular axis. Oestrogens also have a role in epiphyseal closure at puberty, maintaining bone density and, perhaps most surprisingly, in the testis itself. The gene encoding the oestrogen receptor is expressed throughout the testis as is the gene encoding the aromatase enzyme responsible for converting androgens to oestrogen. Consequently, there are high levels of oestrogen present in the testis. This locally produced oestrogen has a role both in the fetal development of the male reproductive system and in the maintenance of normal testicular function in adult men.

Interesting fact

Because the enzyme aromatase is found mainly in adipose tissue, very obese men tend to convert more of their testosterone to oestrogen than lean men. This can lead to significant levels of circulating oestrogens which have feminizing effects, including breast development, decreased facial hair and altered pubic hair distribution. (The male pattern of pubic hair is more of a diamond shape going up to the umbilicus, whereas the female pattern is more triangular with the base of the triangle level with the pubic symphysis.)

Hormone-dependent cancer in men

Prostate cancer is a common condition in older men. The prostate gland is dependent on testosterone for its normal functioning and most prostate cancers are testosterone-dependent, making it a classical example of

Unexpected fracture: 2

Case note: Examination

Mr Smith had rib fractures after a small fall and this suggested that the underlying bones were not healthy. The most likely reason was osteoporosis due to a reduced level of sex steroids. The examination showed small testes, reduced body hair, increased breast tissue, and long arms and legs. These observations are all consistent with decreased androgen activity.

Testosterone is required for male development and bone function. In Mr Smith's case, testosterone deficiency resulted in gynaecomastia, osteoporosis and reduced body hair. The long limbs are due to continuing growth due to delayed fusion of the growth plates, which is controlled by testosterone.

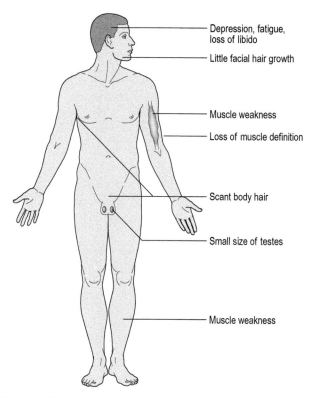

Depression, fatigue, loss of libido

Little facial hair growth

Muscle weakness

Loss of muscle definition

Scant body hair

Small size of testes

Muscle weakness

Figure 8.12 Signs and symptoms of hypogonadism.

a hormone-dependent cancer. As with other hormone-dependent cancers, treatments can aim to block the target hormone's effects on the cancer cells' growth and cell division. Hormone treatment is not usually a first-line treatment option but is used in conjunction with other treatments to shrink the tumour. The aim of treatment is to prevent testosterone from acting on the cancer cells. There are two ways of doing this, either by removing the testosterone itself or by stopping it from acting.

The oldest way of removing the testosterone is to remove the testes: an orchidectomy. However, there are also drug treatments which can stop the production of testosterone by Leydig cells. The most effective treatment is with an LHRH agonist. LHRH is another name for GnRH. We have already noted that this hormone has to be released in a pulsatile fashion in order to be effective at stimulating LH secretion. An LHRH agonist is either given as a long-acting injection or an implant, so that the release of hormone is constant. This constant release very effectively switches off LH and testosterone secretion.

The other treatment is to stop testosterone from acting on prostate cells by using an anti-androgen which blocks testosterone binding to the androgen receptor. An example of this type of drug is cyproterone acetate. Oestrogens are also used as anti-androgenic drugs. These are both taken as daily tablets.

All these treatments have the aim of reducing testosterone effects in the body and so the adverse effects of treatment are related to removal of testosterone: erectile dysfunction and some degree of feminization. They can also cause osteoporosis and mood changes and a significant proportion of men experience 'hot flushes', similar to those experienced by women as a result of oestrogen loss in the menopause. It hardly needs saying that prostate cancer is a serious disorder, with the adverse effects of treatment contributing significantly to the distress caused by the diagnosis itself.

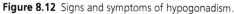

Disorders of male reproduction

Hypogonadism can arise through failure of testicular function (primary hypogonadism), pituitary failure (secondary hypogonadism) or, more rarely, hypothalamic failure (tertiary hypogonadism). The symptoms of hypogonadism are the same, regardless of the cause, with infertility, impotence and loss of male secondary sexual characteristics (Fig. 8.12). There is also a syndrome of partial androgen insensitivity which is considered in more detail in Chapter 10.

Primary hypogonadism

This describes a disorder of testicular function itself, in the presence of normal hypothalamic and pituitary function. Because the normal feedback from testosterone is missing, GnRH and LH/FSH levels are raised, so primary hypogonadism is sometimes called 'hypergonadotropic hypogonadism'. The most common cause of primary hypogonadism is Klinefelter's syndrome, a chromosomal abnormality that results in small testes and failure of secondary sex characteristics. It is discussed in more detail in Chapter 10. Other causes of primary hypogonadism include mumps orchitis, cryptorchidism (failure of testes to descend into scrotum) and testicular damage from radiation or chemotherapy.

Treatment of primary hypogonadism consists of steroid replacement therapy in order to maintain secondary

Case 8.1 — Unexpected fracture: 3

Case note: Investigation

Blood tests revealed:

Luteinizing hormone (LH)	35 U/L (normal <10 U/L)
Follicle stimulating hormone (FSH)	65 U/L (normal <10 U/L)
Testosterone	4 nmol/L (normal 9–41 nmol/L)
Sperm count	Very low

The testis is controlled by LH and FSH. LH stimulates testosterone production from Leydig cells. FSH stimulates the Sertoli cells to initiate and then support the maturation of germ cells into sperm. Mr Smith's results indicate that the testes were abnormal (this is called primary hypogonadism) and that both the Leydig cells and seminiferous tubules were not working.

sex characteristics—normal growth of pubic and axillary hair and sexual function. The infertility resulting from primary hypogonadism is not reversible.

Secondary hypogonadism

Also called hypogonadotropic hypogonadism, secondary hypogonadism is caused by failure of the pituitary gland to secrete appropriate quantities of the gonadotropins, LH and FSH. It is uncommon and usually associated with general hypopituitarism.

Tertiary hypogonadism

Tertiary hypogonadism, the other form of hypogonadotropic hypogonadism, is caused by failure of GnRH secretion from the hypothalamus. The most common cause of disordered GnRH secretion is Kallmann's syndrome, a hereditary disorder that is often associated with anosmia, an impaired sense of smell.

Therapeutic uses of androgens

Testosterone replacement therapy is routinely given to treat the symptoms of hypogonadism, as in the case of Mr Smith. In such situations, testosterone is very helpful in maintaining a normal masculine appearance and in preserving bone health. When testosterone is used in this way there are usually no problems with adverse effects. However, the situation is very different when these steroids are taken for other reasons, usually at high doses (Fig. 8.13).

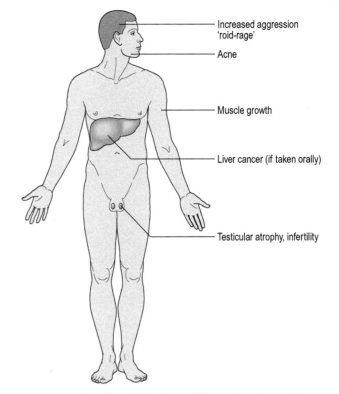

Figure 8.13 Side-effects of abusing anabolic androgenic steroids in men. In women there are additional problems, including the masculinizing effects of these steroids: deepening voice, facial hair growth, acquisition of male body shape, altered serum lipid profile and amenorrhoea.

Case 8.1 — Unexpected fracture: 4

Case note: Diagnosis and treatment

The underlying reason for these findings was Klinefelter's syndrome. This is a common chromosomal abnormality with an incidence of 1 in 500 births. It involves a duplication of the X chromosome resulting in the abnormal karyotype 47XXY.

There is no cure for Klinefelter's syndrome. Mr Smith was infertile for life. However, testosterone replacement was given to improve bone and male development, and to prevent fractures.

Abuse of anabolic androgenic steroids

Anabolic androgenic steroids (AASs) are abused mainly by young men. They may be taken by teenagers who want to improve their body image, by body-builders to increase muscle mass, or by athletes in power sports who will gain an advantage from increased muscle mass, enhanced aggression and, it is believed, improved endurance and faster recovery from injury. Although it may be argued that testosterone is a 'natural substance', when used as a drug of abuse it has a number of serious side-effects, and the synthetic analogues of testosterone, such as tetrahydrogestrinone (THG) and stanozolol, have similar adverse effects. It is simply not possible to separate the 'desirable' anabolic effects from the 'undesirable' androgenic actions of these steroids.

One of the major side-effects of using anabolic steroids is infertility. Synthetic AASs act just like testosterone itself in exerting negative feedback on the hypothalamus and pituitary, inhibiting gonadotropin secretion. This means that the testes will shrink (atrophy) and stop producing both testosterone and sperm. Women who abuse AASs are likely to become masculinized, developing a deep voice and increased body hair (hirsutism), while ceasing menstruation. There are other serious side-effects due to the usual route of administration of these steroids: most androgens are harmful to the liver if taken orally, resulting in a significant risk of liver cancer.

Declining sperm counts

In the second half of the 20th century, a number of studies reported that there was a decline in the average sperm count of men in the developed world. There have also been studies in wildlife populations reporting feminization of male fish, reptiles and some mammalian species, including a report on hermaphrodite polar bears. There is good evidence that the effects seen in wildlife populations are due to chemicals in the environment that have oestrogenic effects. These chemicals include pesticides, various organochlorides and excreted oestrogens in sewage effluent. They are properly classified as 'environmental endocrine disruptors' and have a wide range of effects on different endocrine systems. Almost inevitably, however, those chemicals with oestrogenic actions that cause feminization are termed 'gender benders'. Although the circumstantial evidence appears to be strong, there is presently no direct evidence that these chemicals are also responsible for the reported decline in human sperm counts.

HORMONAL CONTROL OF REPRODUCTION PART II: FEMALE REPRODUCTIVE SYSTEM

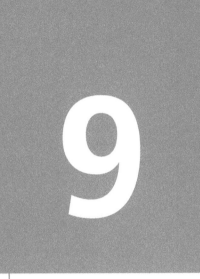

Chapter objectives

After studying this chapter you should be able to:

1. Describe the structure and function of the ovary and outline its relation to the other female reproductive organs.

2. Describe the hormone secretion by the ovary and outline the functions of these hormones.

3. Describe the hormonal control of the menstrual cycle.

4. Outline the major hormonal disorders of the female reproductive system.

5. Explain the hormonal changes that occur in pregnancy.

6. Outline the hormonal control of parturition and lactation.

Introduction

There are some clear similarities between the male and female reproductive systems, but some very obvious differences. In men there is a relatively constant production of gametes, both on a day-to-day basis and throughout adult life, whereas in women there is the production of a single egg each month, which ceases at about the age of 50 years. Although both male and female reproduction are regulated by the same hormones, it is clear that these need to act very differently to coordinate reproductive function in men and women.

Structure of the ovary

The ovaries are the female gonads. They have two main functions: the production of oocytes; and the synthesis of female sex hormones—oestrogens and progestogens. There are two ovaries, lying in the abdomen on either side of the uterus. They are almond-shaped glands, approximately 4 cm long, and are connected to the uterus via the fallopian tubes (Fig. 9.1). The blood supply to the ovaries is from the ovarian arteries which arise directly from the aorta, just beneath the renal arteries. Venous drainage on the right is into the inferior vena cava, and on the left is into the renal vein. This is exactly the same as the venous drainage of the testes.

The ovary contains a number of follicles (Fig. 9.2). The great majority are primordial follicles, the pool of undeveloped oocytes. Unlike the system of gamete production in the male, which is a continuous process throughout life, a woman has only the number of oocytes she is born with. These develop and mature, usually one at a time, during her reproductive life. Typically, there are millions of primordial follicles in the fetal ovary, with about 400 000 at the time of menarche (onset of menstrual bleeding).

Structurally, each primary oocyte is surrounded by a single layer of granulosa cells within a basement membrane. During the reproductive life of a woman, between puberty and menopause, many of these primordial follicles will grow to form mature oocytes, one of which is released at ovulation each month. The development of a primordial follicle into a mature oocyte (Fig. 9.3) takes several months and starts with the process of follicle recruitment: the selection of one primordial follicle for further development. This process is known to be independent of the gonadotropins; recent evidence has implicated the anti-müllerian hormone (see Ch. 10) as an inhibitor of follicular response to FSH, but otherwise little is understood about the process of follicle selection.

As the primordial follicle develops, the single layer of cells around it divides and forms the granulosa cell layer (Fig. 9.3). As the follicle develops further, stromal cells grow around the outside of the follicle to form the theca layer. After ovulation these granulosa and theca cells remain actively secretory and comprise the corpus

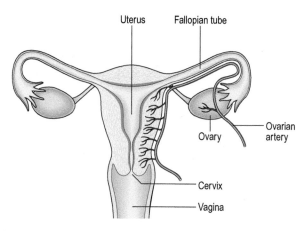

Figure 9.1 The female reproductive system.

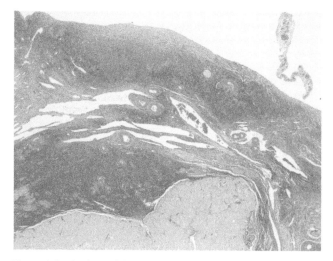

Figure 9.2 Histology of the ovary. (Courtesy of Dr Daniel Berney.)

luteum, 'yellow body', although immediately after ovulation the ruptured follicle fills with blood and appears as a red haemorrhagic body in the ovary. The corpus luteum gradually regresses by a process of apoptosis (this process was originally identified in the ovary) to form a scar-like enclosure called the corpus albicans (Fig. 9.3).

Ovarian hormones

The function of the ovary is two-fold: the production of oocytes and the secretion of hormones. The hormones secreted include the steroids (oestrogens, progesterone and androgens) and the peptides (inhibin, activin and relaxin). Oestrogens and progesterone have an important role in maintaining the endometrial lining of the uterus (see below) and in negative feedback regulation of pituitary hormone release (Fig. 9.4). In contrast to the steroid hormones, the ovarian peptide hormones were discovered more recently and their functions are less well understood. These steroid and peptide hormones are

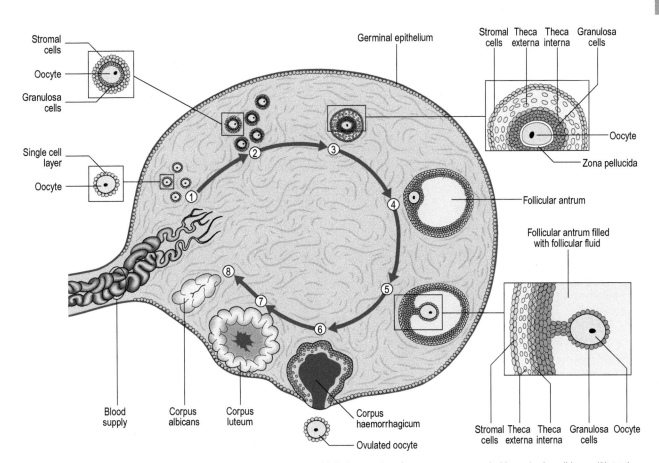

Figure 9.3 Stages of follicular development in the ovary. (1) Primordial follicles consist of an oocyte surrounded by a single cell layer. (2) At the start of follicular development the cells divide to form a stromal layer and surround the granulosa cells. (3) Follicular development continues with the formation of the theca cells, which lie between the granulosa and stromal cells. The oocyte is surrounded by the zona pellucida. (4) The follicular antrum develops, filled with follicular fluid. (5) A mature oocyte: suspended in the follicular fluid, attached by a stalk to the granulosa cell layer. (6) As the follicle ruptures to release the oocyte (the point of ovulation), the antrum fills with blood to form a corpus haemorrhagicum, which develops into the corpus luteum (7). Regression of the corpus luteum leads to the formation of the scar-like corpus albicans (8). The whole cycle shown here takes several months. The developing follicles are not drawn to scale; for comparison, the follicle at stage 2 is around 20μm in diameter whereas the mature follicle at stage 5 is 250 times larger at 5mm, easily visible by eye.

Case 9.1 Imbalanced sex steroids: 1

Case history

Joanna Jones was a 24-year-old woman who presented with increased facial and body hair, acne and irregular periods. The symptoms began when she was about 15 or 16 years old. She noticed coarse hair developing on her cheeks, under her chin, on the front of her chest and around her nipples. Acne appeared on her face and back, and her skin became greasy. Her periods began at the age of 11 years and were always unpredictable, but from age 15 years, she noticed that she would miss one or two periods every 3 months.

Ms Jones' past medical history was unremarkable. She was taking no medications, cigarettes or alcohol. She was a shop assistant and lived with her parents. She had a boyfriend and the couple were planning marriage in the next 12 months and

hoped to start a family. The mother and a maternal aunt had type 2 diabetes mellitus.

On examination, she weighed 85kg and had a height of 163cm, with body mass index of 32kg/m². There was hirsutism over her face, chest, and on her lower body extending from the pubic region to the umbilicus. Her skin was greasy and marked by acne. Fundoscopy, visual fields and eye movements were normal.

1. What is the differential diagnosis?
2. Which tests should be performed to confirm the diagnosis?
3. How will her symptoms and tests guide treatment?
4. Will the couple be infertile?

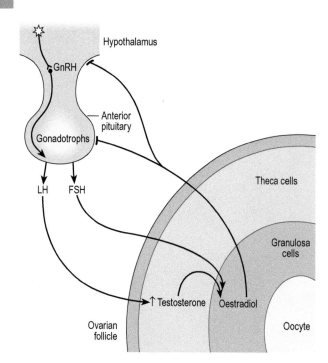

Figure 9.4 Hormonal control of steroidogenesis in the ovarian follicle. The pulsatile release of gonadotropin releasing hormone (GnRH) from the hypothalamus stimulates release of luteinizing hormone (LH) and follicle stimulating hormone (FSH) from the gonadotroph cells of the anterior pituitary. LH receptors are located on the theca cells and LH binds to these receptors, stimulating the secretion of androgens, particularly testosterone. The testosterone is converted to oestradiol in granulosa cells. Levels of the enzyme that catalyse this reaction, aromatase, are increased by the action of FSH on the granulosa cells. Oestradiol exerts a negative feedback effect on the hypothalamus and pituitary.

secreted by the cells of the developing follicle, the theca cells and the granulosa cells (Fig. 9.4), as well as by the corpus luteum.

Transport and metabolism of oestrogen and progesterone

The ovarian steroids are transported in blood bound to carrier proteins. Oestrogen is 60% bound to sex hormone binding globulin (SHBG), with the remaining 40% bound loosely to albumin or in the free form. Progesterone does not have a specific carrier protein but mostly circulates bound to CBG, cortisol binding globulin, and to albumin. The concentration of SHBG in blood is regulated by steroid hormones, being increased by oestrogen and decreased by testosterone. Women therefore have around twice as much SHBG in their blood as men.

In common with other steroids, the ovarian steroids are metabolized in the liver to less active steroids, typically oestrone and oestriol, and excreted in the urine.

A proportion of the oestradiol is conjugated in the liver and excreted in bile salts. There is enterohepatic recycling of steroids by which they are conjugated by the liver and excreted into the gut, where they are de-conjugated and re-absorbed into the circulation. This prolongs the effective half-life of steroids and is particularly important when looking at the contraceptive pill (see Ch. 10).

Oestrogens

The ovaries secrete a range of oestrogens, the female sex steroids, with the principal and most potent of these being oestradiol (Fig. 9.5). There is a close functional interaction between the theca and granulosa cells in the ovary: the theca cells secrete androgens in response to luteinizing hormone (LH) stimulation and these are converted to oestrogens by the adjacent granulosa cells under the control of follicle stimulating hormone (FSH; Fig. 9.5). The ovaries also secrete oestrone and oestriol, although these are also made by conversion of circulating androgens in peripheral tissues.

Cellular actions of oestrogens (Fig. 9.6)

Oestrogens act by binding to a specific oestrogen receptor. There are two forms of this receptor, ERα which is encoded by a gene on chromosome 6, and ERβ, encoded by a gene on chromosome 14. While some tissues contain both forms of the receptors, others express one sub-type preferentially. For example, the α subtype is expressed in the uterus, liver and heart, while the β subtype is found in the ovaries, the central nervous system, the prostate and gastrointestinal tract. Both ER subtypes are members of the family of nuclear receptors. These receptors, like the androgen receptor (Ch. 8) are located in the cytoplasm of the target cell, bound to a chaperone protein called heat shock protein. When oestrogen binds to the receptor, the heat shock protein dissociates and the oestrogen–receptor complex is translocated to the nucleus. The receptor forms dimers, either homodimers (two ERα units joining or two ERβ units joining) or heterodimers (one each α and β unit) and binds to the oestrogen response element on DNA. This complex attracts co-activators which also bind and together permit gene transcription.

Physiological actions of oestrogens

The oestrogens have a wide range of actions in the body, with effects on secondary sex characteristics, metabolism, bone and the brain.

The oestrogens are responsible for the development and maintenance of the secondary sexual characteristics of women, including breast development. In puberty and pregnancy they stimulate growth of the breast ducts and pigmentation of the areoles. They maintain the structure of the vaginal mucosa and stimulate cervical mucus production, maintaining vaginal lubrication. Oestrogens have a permissive role in stimulating growth of the ovarian follicles and promote uterine development, by

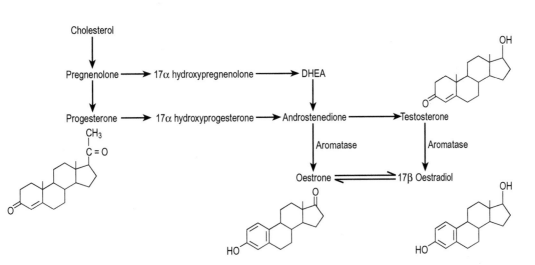

Figure 9.5 Biosynthesis of the major ovarian steroids. Progesterone is both the major secretory product of the corpus luteum and an intermediate in the synthesis of other steroids. Testosterone is synthesized by the theca cells of the follicle and converted into oestradiol by the granulosa cells. DHEA, dehydroepiandrosterone.

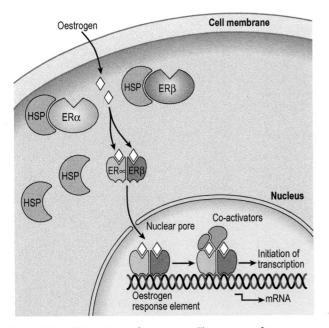

Figure 9.6 Cellular actions of oestrogens. The receptors for oestrogens (ER) are located in the cytoplasm of target cells. In the absence of oestrogen, the receptors are associated with heat shock protein (HSP) which dissociates in the presence of oestrogen. There are two forms of ER, α and β, which can form either homodimers (α-α or β-β) or heterodimers (α-β). When oestrogen binds, the hormone receptor complex moves into the nucleus and binds to the oestrogen response element on DNA. The complex attracts co-activators to form an initiation complex which then allows transcription to proceed.

stimulating endometrial cell proliferation, during the menstrual cycle (see below).

In the brain, oestrogens act to increase libido. It is also thought that they play a role in the process of memory formation and enhance neural repair following injury. Oestrogens are very important for bone health, particularly during the pubertal period when they stimulate closure of the epiphyses in both boys and girls. In addition, oestrogens are thought to be protective against cardiovascular disease. This may be a result of their actions on the liver to reduce circulating cholesterol, but the mechanism of this effect is not fully understood.

Interesting fact

Things are not always as straightforward as they seem. It was observed, some years back, that cows that grazed on fields sprayed with certain pesticides, such as DDT, had lowered fertility rates. The conclusion would seem to be that chemicals like DDT have toxic effects on cows' reproductive systems. However, some of the compounds produced by plants, particularly the isoflavenoids, have weak oestrogenic activity in animals. Plants use these 'phyto-oestrogens' for a variety of functions, including attracting beneficial bacteria to the plants' roots to aid growth. It turned out that chemicals like DDT reduced the plants' ability to attract these bacteria and, in an attempt to attract more, plants such as clover were producing greatly increased amounts of isoflavanoids. In sufficiently large quantities, the weak oestrogenic activity of the ingested flavanoids had a contraceptive effect on the cows, reducing overall fertility. This is a good example of the 'endocrine disruptor' effect of some environmental chemicals, opening up a whole new branch of endocrinology.

Progesterone

Progesterone is secreted principally by the granulosa lutein cells of the corpus luteum which are formed from granulosa cells after the LH surge (see below). Progesterone is the main hormone of pregnancy, and in pregnancy, after week 8, the placenta replaces the corpus luteum as the major source of progesterone. Several steroids have similar properties and are together classified as the 'progestogens'. These include 17α-hydroxyprogesterone and pregnenolone as well as progesterone itself (Fig. 9.5).

Actions of progesterone

Progesterone acts by binding to a specific progesterone receptor which has some similarities with the glucocorticoid receptor. For example, mifepristone, which is used to induce early abortion, binds to both the progesterone and glucocorticoid receptor. There are two isoforms of the progesterone receptor encoded by the same gene, but with different start sites for transcription, hence the increased size of PR-B compared with PR-A. Expression of the progesterone receptor is regulated by oestrogens, while progesterone has an important effect, mediated by PR-A, in inhibiting the proliferative actions of oestrogen. For this reason progesterones are nearly always given in addition to oestrogen therapy, for example in the oral contraceptive pill and in hormone replacement therapy (see Ch. 10).

The main action of progesterone is in the maintenance of pregnancy. Progesterone is responsible for maintaining the structure of the uterus to allow implantation of the embryo, and has an essential role in pregnancy. Blocking progesterone synthesis or action is an effective method for terminating a pregnancy. Progesterone is believed to be a thermogenic steroid, acting to raise body temperature. This property may be exploited in determining a woman's fertile period each month, as there is a small but fairly reliable rise in body temperature, which coincides with increased progesterone secretion following ovulation (see Fig. 9.7D).

Androgen secretion by the ovaries

It may seem surprising to read that the ovary produces androgens, the classical male sex steroids, but these hormones have important functions in women. First, they are essential in the production of oestrogens: the enzyme aromatase converts androgens to oestrogens in both the ovary and adipose tissues (Fig. 9.5). Second, androgens are responsible for the development and maintenance of pubic and axillary hair, and also have an important role in controlling sex drive (libido). The most potent androgen in women, as in men, is testosterone. Much of the circulating testosterone in women comes directly from the ovaries, but the rest is produced by conversion of adrenal androgens (see Ch. 6). The normal circulating concentration of testosterone in adult women is between 1.0 and 3.0 nmol/L, compared with a range of 9–41 nmol/L in men. However, the amount of bio-available testosterone is considerably lower than this in women as they have higher levels of the plasma binding protein, sex hormone binding globulin (SHBG), than men. There are also less potent androgens produced by the ovaries and adrenal,

such as androstenedione and dehydroepiandrosterone (DHEA) that contribute significantly to the total amount of circulating androgen. Excessive androgen production by the ovaries (or adrenals) causes a degree of masculinization and disruption of the normal menstrual cycle. This is described in more detail below in the section on polycystic ovarian syndrome.

Case 9.1 Imbalanced sex steroids: 2

Case note: Differential diagnosis

Joanna's symptoms suggest a disruption of the sex steroid endocrinology. Such diseases can be classified into: excess male hormones or reduced female hormones.

The causes of reduced female hormones can be further separated into diseases of the pituitary/hypothalamus or ovarian failure. There were no symptoms or signs of pituitary or hypothalamic disease (e.g. a visual field defect) or of ovarian failure (e.g. flushing).

The symptoms suggested an excess of male hormones. The commonest cause of this is polycystic ovary syndrome. Rare causes include androgen secreting ovarian or adrenal tumours, or the genetic condition congenital adrenal hyperplasia (see Ch. 6). For every 100 patients with Joanna's symptoms, 98 will have polycystic ovary syndrome and only 2% will suffer from one of the other conditions.

Which tests would you perform to confirm the diagnosis?

Ovarian peptide hormones

Regulatory peptides, inhibin and activin, produced by the Sertoli cells in the testis, are also produced in women, but in the ovaries. In addition, the ovaries produce a third peptide hormone, relaxin.

Inhibin

Inhibin was coined as a term in the 1930s, but the peptide hormone was isolated only in the 1980s. It is a glycoprotein, secreted by the granulosa and theca cells of the developing follicle, and has a role in inhibiting FSH secretion. It has been suggested that inhibin may have a role in follicle selection. Inhibin levels may also be an early marker of the onset of menopause.

Activin

Activin is a member of the transforming growth factor-β (TGF-β) peptide family. It was also isolated in the 1980s as a potential reproductive hormone but is now thought to have a more significant role in the inflammatory response. High concentrations of activin are also produced by the endometrium and have a role in the development of the endometrium during the menstrual cycle. Clinically, activin may have a role as a prognostic indicator in women undergoing treatment to stimulate ovulation, as part of assisted conception.

Relaxin

Relaxin was first identified in the 1920s. It is now known that there are seven members of the relaxin family of peptides, with a range of different roles. Relaxin stimulates follicular development and oocyte maturation, and may have a role in implantation of the embryo. It is known to have an important role in parturition and has a number of other effects outside the reproduction system, including an antifibrotic action in wound healing.

Hormonal regulation of ovarian function

Ovarian function is controlled by the two gonadotropins, luteinizing hormone (LH) and follicle stimulating hormone (FSH), secreted by the gonadotroph cells of the anterior pituitary under the control of gonadotropin releasing hormone (GnRH) from the hypothalamus (Fig. 9.4). In women, as in men, release of these hormones is pulsatile, with both the amplitude and the frequency of pulses varying through the menstrual cycle.

The basic principle of the hormonal control of ovarian function is simple: the hormones do what their names suggest. FSH stimulates the growth of the developing follicle, and LH stimulates steroid production by the corpus luteum and the developing follicle. The cellular mechanism of action of LH and FSH in the ovary is essentially the same as in the testis (see Ch. 8). A surge in the production of LH is responsible for stimulating ovulation. There is only one small complication: although LH stimulates androgen secretion by the follicle, it is under the control of FSH that this is converted to oestrogen.

Hormone-dependent cancer in women

Oestrogens have strongly proliferative effects in breast tissue and in the endometrial lining of the uterus. So it is not surprising that, in both these tissues, oestrogens may also act as tumour promoters, stimulating the growth of cancer cells. It is worth noting that oestrogens do not cause the damage that gives rise to tumour cells, but when mutations of DNA occur and tumour cells develop, then oestrogen can stimulate the growth of these cells. Oestrogen receptors are routinely measured in breast cancer biopsies and about half of all breast cancers are oestrogen receptor positive. Of these ER positive tumours, about 70% will respond to treatment with the anti-oestrogen tamoxifen. If progesterone receptors are also present then this increases the response rate slightly to about 80%.

An increased risk of breast and endometrial cancer is one of the adverse effects of taking hormone replacement therapy containing oestrogen. In order to minimize the risk, progesterone is added to both HRT and the contraceptive pill, as progesterone opposes the proliferative effects of oestrogens. Selective oestrogen receptor modulators are used to treat oestrogen-dependent cancers (Box 9.1).

The menstrual cycle

This is the term given to the cycle of hormonal and other physiological changes that commences with the shedding of the endometrium (the uterine lining) and includes the release of a mature oocyte from the ovarian follicle. It is the basic unit of reproductive time in women, producing a single mature germ cell each month, and is essential for understanding the reproductive process (Fig. 9.7). The average menstrual cycle lasts for 28 days—hence the term 'menstrual', meaning 'monthly'. Cycle length is usually fairly regular for an individual, but can vary between women over a considerable range, with most women having a cycle between 21 and 35 days long. In puberty

Box 9.1 Selective oestrogen receptor modulators (SERMs)

There is a range of drugs available which modify oestrogen actions in a tissue-specific manner. These are called SERMs and may act to inhibit oestrogen actions in some tissues while stimulating oestrogen receptors in other tissues. They are partial agonists and partial antagonists at the oestrogen receptor. The question of whether a drug acts as an agonist or an antagonist in a specific tissue depends partly on the predominant ER subtype expressed in that tissue and partly on the nuclear factors, co-activators and co-repressors present in the cells.

The most well-known SERM is tamoxifen, which is used clinically to block the actions of oestrogen on breast cancer cells and so to inhibit growth of breast cancers. Tamoxifen has beneficial effects on bone in postmenopausal women and also acts on the liver to decrease circulating cholesterol. However, prolonged use is associated with an increased risk of endometrial cancer as tamoxifen has agonist effects on ER in the uterus.

Clomiphene, another SERM, acts to block the negative feedback effects of oestradiol at the hypothalamus and pituitary and so causes an increase in FSH levels. It is used to stimulate ovulation in anovulatory women and is particularly used in polycystic ovarian syndrome. Like tamoxifen, it stimulates uterine ER and so increases the risk of endometrial cancer.

Phyto-oestrogens, which are naturally occurring oestrogens found in plants, also appear to act as SERMs. The discovery that drugs can be developed with selective actions in certain tissues gives rise to the hope for a new form of postmenopausal HRT that has all the benefits of oestrogen itself, but without the risks of breast and endometrial cancer.

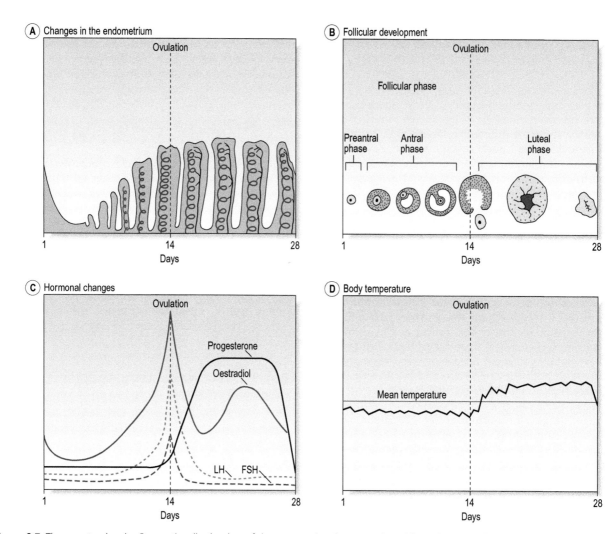

Figure 9.7 The menstrual cycle. Conventionally, the days of the menstrual cycle are numbered from the onset of menstruation (day 1). Ovulation occurs on day 14 in the standard 28-day cycle. The duration of the proliferative phase (the interval from the onset of menstruation to ovulation) is variable and ovulation does not always occur on day 14. However, there is little variation in the length of the secretory phase. (A) Changes in the endometrium during the menstrual cycle. (B) Stages of follicular development during the menstrual cycle. (C) Hormonal changes during the menstrual cycle; the peak in oestradiol immediately precedes ovulation. (D) Changes in body temperature during the menstrual cycle. Basal body temperature rises, under the influence of progesterone, after ovulation and remains higher than mean during the secretory phase, falling to slightly below mean temperature with the onset of menstruation.

and in the perimenopausal period, the cycle length may be considerably longer. The variation in cycle length is almost always due to variations in the follicular/proliferative phase.

There are several phases to the menstrual cycle that describe changes to both the ovary and the uterus.

The menstrual phase

In most numbering conventions, day 1 of the menstrual cycle is the day on which endometrial shedding starts. For a woman it is the first day of her monthly 'period'. The endometrial lining of the uterus, which has developed during the previous cycle, is shed through the vagina together with a small amount of blood. This vaginal bleeding usually lasts between 4 and 7 days. There are several disorders associated with menstruation, with perhaps the commonest being *dysmenorrhoea*, a term applied to the painful abdominal cramps experienced by many women during their period. This vasospasm is probably due to the high levels of prostaglandin production by the endometrium.

The follicular phase (also called the proliferative phase)

The proliferative phase describes the changes that occur in the uterus while the follicle is maturing in the ovary, prior to ovulation. Under the influence of oestrogens secreted by the follicle before ovulation, the endometrium proliferates and develops a rich blood supply. This process is called 'decidualization' of the endometrium. During this phase, the selected follicle undergoes the last stages of its maturation within the ovary prior to release of the oocyte. Gonadotropin secretion from the pituitary stimulates oestrogen synthesis by the developing follicle.

Usually, increasing oestrogen levels would inhibit further gonadotropin release, but this negative feedback mechanism is suspended during the late follicular phase, and there is a peak in LH secretion which immediately precedes ovulation (Fig. 9.7C). At this point, immediately pre-ovulation, the follicle is pressed against the wall of the ovary forming a bulge called the stigma.

The LH surge and ovulation

This LH surge has a number of effects on granulosa cells and on the surrounding structures: first it rapidly down-regulates CYP 19 expression in granulosa cells and so

blocks the formation of oestrogens. This removes the negative feedback effect of oestrogens on the hypothalamus and pituitary and allows LH secretion to increase. The increased LH stimulates the release of prostaglandins and inflammatory cytokines which lead to a rupture of the stromal cells and the germinal epithelium of the ovary. This allows release of the oocyte from the follicle.

LH also causes breakdown of the basal lamina surrounding the follicle. Finally, it stimulates the expression in granulosa cells of the enzymes of steroidogenesis which were previously only expressed in the theca cells: CYP11A1 (cholesterol side chain cleavage) and 3β-HSD. Together with increased StAR expression, these changes allow the granulosa cells to begin secreting progesterone and to form the basis of the corpus luteum.

The luteal phase (also called the secretory phase)

The luteal phase is dominated by the actions of progesterone. After ovulation, the ruptured follicle from which the ovum was released forms a corpus haemorrhagicum,

---

Case 9.1 Imbalanced sex steroids: 3

Case note: Investigations

Joanna had a morning blood sample taken on day 21 of her menstrual cycle and an ultrasonographic scan of the ovaries was performed.

Prolactin	365 mU/L (normal <400 mU/L)
LH/FSH	18/4 U/L (normal <10 U/L)
Oestradiol	639 pmol/L (normal luteal phase, 400–1200 pmol/L)
Progesterone	<3 nmol/L (normal luteal phase >30 nmol/L)
Cortisol	314 nmol/L (normal, 200–600 nmol/L)
Testosterone	2.1 nmol/L (normal >3 nmol/L)
SHBG	25 nmol/L (normal, 20–120 nmol/L)
Androstenedione	17.2 nmol/L (normal <8 nmol/L)
Dehydroepiandrosterone sulphate (DHEAS)	6.1 μmol/L (normal <6.8 μmol/L)
17α-Hydroxyprogesterone	3.7 nmol/L (normal <10 nmol/L)
Ultrasonography	Multiple cysts in both ovaries with increased stroma between the cysts.

The prolactin and oestradiol levels were normal, which made a pituitary or hypothalamic cause for her disease unlikely. The normal 17α-hydroxyprogesterone concentration made congenital adrenal hyperplasia less likely. Virilizing adrenal

or ovarian tumours often produce high serum testosterone levels (frequently >0.5 nmol/L), making these diagnoses less likely. Cushing's syndrome is due to an excess of cortisol, and adrenal production of androgens may also be increased. Thus, Cushing's syndrome may cause similar symptoms (but usually gives a thin skin rather than a thick skin). Here, the normal serum cortisol level made this diagnosis less likely.

These results are common for polycystic ovary syndrome. The male hormones are either high (androstenedione) or in the upper part of the normal range (testosterone and DHEAS), and the SHBG concentration is low. SHBG circulates with testosterone and inactivates it. A low serum SHBG level exacerbates the imbalance of male hormones. The LH/FSH ratio is characteristically higher in polycystic ovary syndrome, for unknown reasons.

The ultrasonographic appearances supported the diagnosis. However, ultrasonography of the ovaries is not a reliable diagnostic tool in polycystic ovary syndrome. This is because about 20% of healthy women with no symptoms of endocrine disease show multiple cysts on ultrasonography and do not have polycystic ovary syndrome.

The cause of polycystic ovary syndrome is unknown, but it is linked to increased body weight, insulin resistance (presumably causing a thickened skin) and a risk of diabetes mellitus. The working definition of polycystic ovary syndrome is the presence of symptoms of androgen excess with raised serum androgen levels *and* the exclusion of other diseases.

How will Joanna's symptoms and test results guide treatment?

formed by bleeding into the ruptured follicle. This matures to form the corpus luteum which has a limited life of around 14 days (unless the ovum is fertilized, in which case the corpus luteum persists). In the absence of a fertilized ovum the corpus luteum degenerates—a process termed 'luteolysis'—and stops secreting progesterone. It is this decrease in progesterone secretion that causes the breakdown of the endometrium and the start of menstruation.

The luteal phase is also referred to as the 'secretory phase'. This refers both to the secretion of progesterone from the corpus luteum and to the secretion of a clear fluid by the endometrium during this phase.

Interesting fact

Only higher primates have menstrual cycles with regular bleeding. Lower mammals have an oestrous cycle that does not include menstruation; instead, the uterine lining is broken down and resorbed. The oestrous cycle is most easily understood as a cycle of sexual receptivity. The word 'oestrous' comes from the Greek for the 'gadfly', suggesting the frenzied activity exhibited by some mammals when 'in heat'. Many mammals are 'continuous cyclers', like humans, whereas others have seasonal oestrous cycles with only one (cows and pigs) or two (dogs) cycles per year.

Disorders of the menstrual cycle

Amenorrhoea is either the absence of menarche in a girl by the age of 16 years, known as primary amenorrhoea, or the failure of three or more menstrual periods in succession in a woman who previously had an established cycle, known as secondary amenorrhoea. Delayed puberty and primary amenorrhoea are discussed in detail in Chapter 10, so we will focus here on secondary amenorrhoea, following established menstruation.

There are many causes of secondary amenorrhoea, but the commonest by far is pregnancy. The first investigation to be carried out in a woman who presents with amenorrhoea should always be a pregnancy test. Other causes of amenorrhoea can be broadly divided into ovarian failure, pituitary failure and hypothalamic failure, although amenorrhoea may also result from other endocrine disorders such as adrenal disorders. Do not be confused by the classification of amenorrhoea, which is different from that of other endocrine disorders, due to the fact that menstruation only starts at menarche. The adrenal gland, for example, needs to function normally from birth, so primary adrenal failure refers to a disorder of adrenal function originating in the adrenal gland itself. With amenorrhoea, the most significant issue is whether the system has ever worked properly, so primary ovarian failure refers to the situation where menarche has never occurred, regardless of the cause.

Hypothalamic causes

This is one of the commonest causes of non-pregnant amenorrhoea, and is the underlying problem in about one-third of cases. Hypothalamic causes include the amenorrhoea associated with excessive exercise and with eating disorders. In these disorders, there is severe disruption of the hypothalamic secretion of GnRH, which leads to failure of pituitary LH and FSH secretion, and then to impaired ovarian function. It is likely that a decrease in body mass and in the proportion of body fat may contribute to the impaired GnRH secretion, and it is thought that leptin may be the link between body fat and hypothalamic function (see Ch. 13).

Pituitary causes

Hyperprolactinaemia accounts for approximately one-third of cases of non-pregnant amenorrhoea. It has been suggested that up to 5% of the adult population have an undiagnosed pituitary micro-prolactinoma, producing excessive amounts of prolactin. Prolactin is well known to cause disturbances of the menstrual cycle because it inhibits the pulsatile secretion of hypothalamic GnRH. In lactating women the high levels of circulating prolactin can be a useful, although not totally reliable, form of contraception. Hyperprolactinaemia is commonly treated with a dopamine agonist, such as bromocriptine or cabergoline.

Any disorder causing functional disturbance of anterior pituitary function will result in impaired gonadotropin secretion (see Ch. 4).

Ovarian causes

Premature ovarian failure

Ovarian failure at the appropriate time is called menopause and will be considered in the next chapter. Premature ovarian failure, which is also called premature menopause, is diagnosed when ovarian failure occurs before the age of 40 years. This is not a common disorder. There is often a genetic cause, such as Turner's syndrome, which is characterized by the absence of one X chromosome (see Ch. 10). It occurs in around 1 in 3000 female babies. Other causes include autoimmune destruction of the ovary, which is usually associated with other autoimmune disease, such as Graves' disease.

Polycystic ovarian syndrome (PCOS)

This syndrome is a common cause of amenorrhoea, accounting for up to 20% of cases. It is characterized by excessive androgen secretion, which is not a result of congenital adrenal hyperplasia or other cause. The excessive androgen secretion is often the problem that causes the patient to visit her doctor. She may notice increased facial and body hair (Box 9.2), greasy skin and acne as well as irregular monthly periods (Fig. 9.8). Ultrasonographic examination of the

Box 9.2 Hirsutism

Hirsutism is the term used to describe the growth of facial hair and excess body hair in women. The hair is commonly seen on the upper lip and chin, on the chest, abdomen, thighs and forearms. The extent of body hair on a woman is familial and the perception of body hair on a woman is culturally determined, so what is considered normal for one woman may be considered hirsute by another. Hirsutism may reflect an underlying endocrine abnormality, such as congenital adrenal hyperplasia, but this is rare. A change in body hair in an adult woman may reflect the development of polycystic ovarian syndrome, which is relatively common, but in the great majority of women, body and facial hair is quite normal. Because of the cultural taboos around the issue of body and facial hair, most hirsute women choose cosmetic treatment to either remove or bleach the hair so that it is less noticeable.

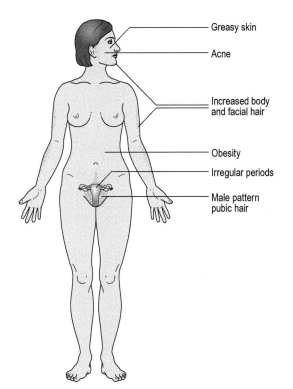

Figure 9.8 Common features of polycystic ovarian syndrome (PCOS).

Greasy skin

Acne

Increased body and facial hair

Obesity

Irregular periods

Male pattern pubic hair

ovaries reveals enlarged ovaries containing numerous cysts, from 2 to 8 mm in size. However, ovarian cysts are very common and may be present in 20% of women who have no menstrual irregularity and who do not have PCOS. PCOS cannot be seen as a purely ovarian disorder: type 2 diabetes mellitus is a common finding in women with PCOS and 50% of women with PCOS are clinically obese.

Although women with PCOS usually experience menstrual irregularities and thus reduced fertility, many still ovulate occasionally. There is a great variation between individuals in the degree of reduced fertility caused by PCOS.

The treatment for this disorder is generally just to manage the symptoms, as there is no cure at present. The mainline treatment is to use synthetic oestrogens and progestogens (as in the contraceptive pill) to reduce LH and FSH secretion and ovarian steroid secretion. This has the effect of decreasing the amount of androgen produced and so of reversing the effects of excessive androgen secretion. In some cases an androgen receptor antagonist may also be used.

Case 9.1 Imbalanced sex steroids: 4

Case note: Treatment

How will Joanna Jones' symptoms, test results and future plans guide treatment?

There is no cure for polycystic ovary syndrome, because the cause is unknown. It is not even clear that the ovaries are the sole source of the increased levels of androgens. Adrenal and ovarian vein catheter studies have shown androgen production from both the ovaries and the adrenal glands. This makes surgical treatment unrealistic. Nearly all patients find hirsutism and acne very distressing. These problems can be controlled with a combination of drugs: oestradiol to counterbalance the androgens, and an androgen blocker or inhibitor to lower the effect of the androgens on the skin. However, the couple desire a family and this combination of treatments will act as an oral contraceptive and may harm sexual development in a male fetus. So, if pregnancy is the main goal, other treatments will be needed.

Interesting fact

Some years ago, a lot of interest was aroused by studies that seemed to show that groups of women living together, for example at boarding school, in religious institutions or in prisons, tended to have synchronized menstrual cycles. Subsequent studies have not supported this idea and have shown that, generally, synchronization does not occur in women, although there is good evidence for it in other species. Despite this, there has been an increased interest in the proposed mechanism of synchronization: pheromones. A pheromone is a chemical signal produced by one individual that causes behavioural changes in another without consciously being detected by the senses. Pheromones are therefore quite different from scents, which are detected by the olfactory apparatus. It has been known for some time that pheromones are important modulators of animal behaviour, but there is increasing evidence that there are also human pheromones. Their role remains a matter of speculation.

Case 9.1 Imbalanced sex steroids: 5

Case note: Fertility
Will the couple be infertile?

Joanna was not ovulating regularly, as her menstrual cycle was not regular and the progesterone level taken on day 21 of the cycle was undetectable, indicating an infertile cycle. So it is likely that Joanna will have reduced fertility. However, fertility is difficult to predict as some patients with severe polycystic ovary syndrome still ovulate intermittently. Thus, if the couple do not desire pregnancy, they should be advised to use contraception.

In order to induce ovulation, Joanna will need a diet and exercise programme to improve her weight and insulin resistance. The drug metformin lowers insulin resistance (see Ch. 11) and may improve ovulation. Clomiphene (a partial oestrogen receptor agonist) is effective when used together with metformin in stimulating ovulation. It is likely that the couple will be able to conceive with treatment.

The endocrinology of pregnancy

The placenta

Pregnancy results when the released ovum is fertilized by a spermatozoon. Fertilization may occur in either the fallopian tubes or the uterus. The conceptus becomes embedded in the endometrial lining of the uterus and establishes a blood supply via the placenta. The fetus and the mother are genetically distinct individuals and are linked by the placenta, which is maternal tissue, not fetal tissue. The placenta provides the blood supply to the fetus and so regulates the supply of nutrients to the fetus. The placenta is also the major endocrine tissue of pregnancy. It sends hormonal signals to the corpus luteum, preventing luteal regression and maintaining progesterone and oestrogen secretion for the early part of pregnancy. It also metabolizes maternal hormones and controls the endocrine environment of the developing fetus.

Hormone secretion by the placenta

The major hormone produced by the developing placenta in the first weeks of gestation (pregnancy) is human chorionic gonadotropin (hCG) (see Fig. 9.11). hCG is structurally very similar to LH and has an important role in maintaining luteal function and preventing the normal regression of the corpus luteum which ends an infertile menstrual cycle. Box 9.3 outlines how methods of detecting hCG have been developed over the years in pregnancy testing.

The placenta secretes a range of steroids, but it differs from other steroid-secreting tissues because it does not use StAR protein to transport cholesterol across the mitochondrial membrane. After about 8 weeks' gestation the placenta takes over from the corpus luteum as the major source of progesterone, although the corpus luteum persists throughout pregnancy. The placental secretion of progesterone increases throughout pregnancy and is essential to maintain pregnancy. It is thought that progesterone acts to keep the myometrium (the muscular lining of the uterus) in a relaxed state, preventing contractions and expulsion of the fetus. This is partly achieved by inhibiting oxytocin receptor expression. Progesterone may also have a role in appetite and energy regulation.

Other steroids produced by the placenta include the oestrogens—oestrone, oestradiol and oestriol—levels of which all increase throughout pregnancy (Fig. 9.11). This is the result of a complicated interaction with the adrenal gland of the fetus, with early steroid products from the placenta being metabolized by the fetal adrenal gland and finally converted to oestrogens by the placenta (see below).

The placenta also secretes testosterone, which increases in concentration during pregnancy, reaching 10 times pre-pregnancy levels at term, as well as a placental lactogen (hPL, also known as human chorionic somatomammotropin, hCS), which stimulates breast development during pregnancy. hPL is closely related to growth hormone and prolactin and also acts to antagonize the effects of insulin, which may have the effect of increasing the supply of nutrients to the fetus. The secretion of hPL increases throughout pregnancy. Late in pregnancy, the placenta also produces CRH, usually a hypothalamic hormone, which has a role in signalling the end of pregnancy (see below).

Interesting fact

The word placenta comes from the Latin meaning 'flat cake'. This etymology is taken literally in the practise of 'placentophagy' (yes, eating one's own placenta). Placentophagy is common in mammals and may have a role in ensuring contraction of the uterus due to the high prostaglandin content. In humans, placentophagy is practised in some cultures but has been increasingly advocated in Europe and the USA as a natural protection against postnatal depression due to the high oestrogen content of placental tissue. There is no evidence to support this practice. There are even recipes on the web for cooking placenta, although true aficionados claim that, for maximum benefit, it should be eaten raw.

The feto–placental unit

The developing fetus is able to produce a range of its own steroid hormones. It is not autonomous, however, and there is a significant interaction between the fetus

Box 9.3 Pregnancy testing

Detection of hCG is the basis of all pregnancy tests. As hCG is normally produced only during pregnancy, it is a reliable and specific indicator of pregnancy. Although it is a fairly large peptide hormone, sufficient hCG is excreted in urine to be detectable by a variety of methods.

Old-fashioned pregnancy testing (Fig. 9.9)

The first pregnancy tests were bioassays for hCG. At first mice were used: groups of five immature female mice were injected with urine then killed some days later. Their ovaries and uterus were inspected, with 'enlargement' confirming the pregnancy. This used large numbers of mice and was fairly unreliable.

In the mid-20th century (1930s–1960s) a simpler bioassay was developed. This was based on the observation that the female *Xenopus* toad (*Xenopus laevis*) would ovulate within 12 h after exposure to hCG. Colonies of these toads were kept in pregnancy testing laboratories, injected with urine samples and checked for ovulation. Ovulation is not easy to miss in a *Xenopus* toad. This test was nearly 100% reliable, the results were available the next day, and the method had the advantage of re-usable toads. It did take a lot of worms, however, to keep the colonies going.

Modern pregnancy testing kit (Fig. 9.10)

The *Xenopus* colonies gradually fell into disuse as more sophisticated immunoassay methods were developed. Modern pregnancy testing kits use a sensitive immunoassay which can detect hCG from about 10 days after conception. The assay uses a colour-change reaction to indicate whether hCG is detected or not. The great advantage of this method is that it can be carried out conveniently at home.

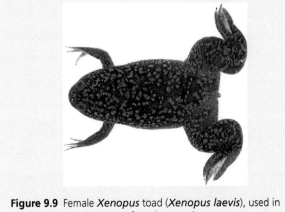

Figure 9.9 Female *Xenopus* toad (*Xenopus laevis*), used in pregnancy tests (courtesy of Xenbase.org).

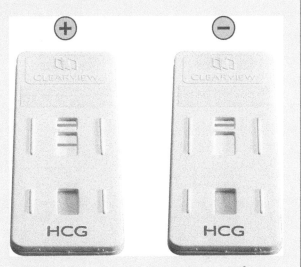

Figure 9.10 Modern pregnancy testing kit. (Clearview® HCG Pregnancy Test, courtesy of Unipath Limited).

---

and the placenta (Fig. 9.12). As we have seen above, the placenta has a great capacity for steroid synthesis. It produces a range of steroids, such as pregnenolone and progesterone, which are conveyed to the fetus where the fetal adrenal converts them into the glucocorticoids, cortisol and corticosterone, and also into the hormone precursors, dehydroepiandrosterone sulphate (DHEAS) and 16-hydroxydehydroepiandrosterone (16-OH-DHEAS). These two steroids are transported back to the placenta where they form the substrate for placental oestrogen synthesis. Hence, the formation of oestrogens in the placenta is a three-stage process: placental synthesis of progesterone and pregnenolone, fetal conversion of these steroids to DHEAS and 16-OH-DHEAS and finally, placental conversion of these steroids into oestrogens.

The placenta also contains high levels of 11 beta hydroxysteroid dehydrogenase, which prevents maternal cortisol from entering the fetal circulation (see below).

Non-placental hormones and binding proteins in pregnancy

In addition to the hormones secreted by the placenta during pregnancy, there are other major effects on the endocrine system (Fig. 9.11). Thyroid hormone secretion increases during the first trimester of pregnancy and then reaches a plateau, although thyroid hormone binding globulin (THBG) concentration increases as well, so there is no overall change in free thyroxine levels. Cortisol secretion increases throughout pregnancy, reaching three times the pre-pregnancy level at term, although adrenocorticotropic hormone (ACTH) secretion is unchanged. From the anterior pituitary, LH and FSH levels are very low throughout pregnancy, while the level of thyroid stimulating hormone (TSH) dips during the first trimester and then returns to pre-pregnancy levels. Growth hormone secretion is unchanged, but prolactin levels rise progressively throughout pregnancy.

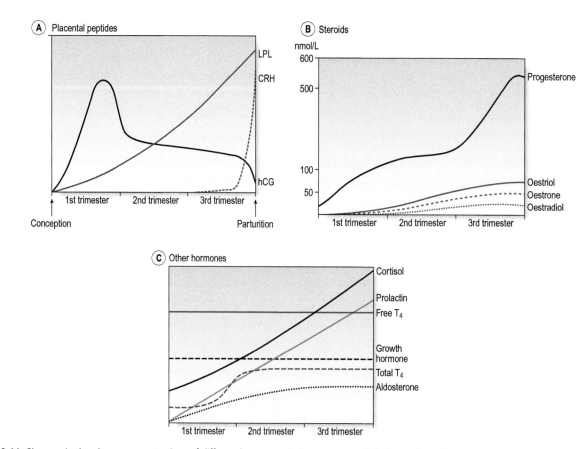

Figure 9.11 Changes in the plasma concentrations of different hormones during pregnancy. (A) Placental peptides. Human chorionic gonadotropin (hCG) is the major peptide secreted in the first trimester, and peaks at around 10 weeks' gestation. Levels of human placental lactogen (hPL), in contrast, rise gradually throughout gestation, peaking just before parturition. Corticotropin releasing hormone (CRH) is the third placental peptide, and is a hormone of late pregnancy, increasing only about 3 weeks before parturition. (B) Steroid hormones. Progesterone is the major steroid hormone of pregnancy, with levels increasing throughout gestation, peaking just before parturition and falling sharply afterwards. Of the other steroids, oestriol is the major oestrogen. Levels of all the oestrogens rise gradually during pregnancy. Testosterone concentration, not shown here, also increases throughout pregnancy. (C) Other hormones. Levels of the adrenal hormones, cortisol and aldosterone, increase during pregnancy, with aldosterone reaching a plateau during the third trimester. Total thyroxine concentration increases during the first trimester, although there is no change in free T4 or free T3. Levels of prolactin, from the anterior pituitary, increase throughout pregnancy, but there is no change in growth hormone secretion.

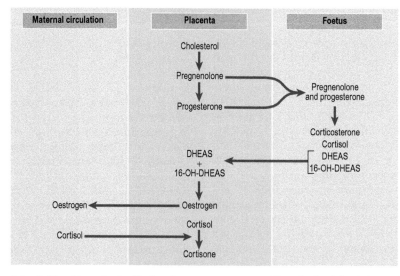

Figure 9.12 The feto–placental unit. Steroids synthesized in the placenta are transported into the fetal circulation and metabolized by the fetal adrenal. Some of these steroids return to the placenta where they undergo further metabolism and enter the maternal circulation. The placenta also inactivates cortisol to prevent fetal exposure to high levels of glucocorticoids.

It is increasingly apparent that events that occur *in utero*, while the fetus is developing, have an effect on health much later in life. This is known as 'fetal programming'. For example, it is known that the placenta has a high expression of 11 beta hydroxysteroid dehydrogenase (11β-HSD), the enzyme which converts the active glucocorticoid cortisol to the inactive cortisone. It appears that this enzyme has an important role in protecting the fetus from high maternal glucocorticoid levels. People whose mothers were treated during pregnancy with synthetic glucocorticoids (such as dexamethasone) which are not inactivated by 11β-HSD during pregnancy, have a higher risk of developing a number of disorders as adults, including hypertension, type II diabetes and an impaired stress response.

Endocrine control of parturition

The signals that initiate parturition (labour) in humans are not well understood. Several hormones are known to be involved, including corticotropin releasing hormone (CRH), which is secreted by the placenta from about 20 days before parturition starts. A decline in progesterone concentration is also involved, as parturition can be initiated by giving the progesterone antagonist RU486. The ovarian peptide hormone, relaxin, has an important role in parturition, promoting cervical ripening. This is the process of growth and softening of the cervix, allowing delivery of the fetus.

In hospital, labour can be induced artificially by the administration of vaginal prostaglandins and injections of oxytocin. However, an increase in oxytocin concentration does not usually occur before the onset of parturition and so does not appear normally to be responsible for initiating labour. Oxytocin is probably more important for coordinating contraction of the myometrium, as levels rise rapidly *during* parturition. Prostaglandins are an important part of the onset of labour as they cause 'ripening' and dilation of the cervix.

It is now thought that the most important signal for labour to start is the increase in corticotropin releasing hormone (CRH) activity in the late stages of pregnancy. This rise is a signal for increased prostaglandin synthesis. However, the onset of parturition is more complex than an increase in the level of a single hormone, and it is clear that there is an interaction between many different hormonal signals.

Lactation

During pregnancy, there is an interaction between several different hormones to stimulate breast development (Fig. 9.13). These include progesterone, human placental lactogen (hPL), prolactin, insulin and cortisol. However,

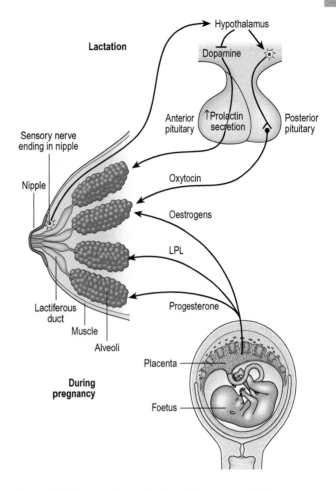

Figure 9.13 Hormonal control of breast development during pregnancy and lactation. During pregnancy, hormones from the placenta, including human placental lactogen (hPL), progesterone and oestrogens, act on the breast and stimulate proliferation of the alveolar tissue in preparation for lactation. The oestrogens prevent lactation from occurring during pregnancy. After parturition, when the influence of the placenta is removed, suckling of the baby stimulates the release of prolactin from the anterior pituitary, thereby stimulating milk formation, and release of oxytocin from the posterior pituitary, causing contraction of the smooth muscle around the alveoli and expelling milk from the breast.

the high oestrogen levels seen during pregnancy put a 'brake' on lactation. This brake is removed by delivery of the baby, which results in a rapid decrease of oestrogen levels and the onset of lactation, mostly under the control of prolactin. Suckling of the baby at the nipple stimulates the release of prolactin from the anterior pituitary and of oxytocin from the posterior pituitary. While prolactin stimulates milk formation, oxytocin stimulates the milk 'let down' reflex by causing contraction of the smooth muscle around the alveoli (milk ducts).

HORMONAL CONTROL OF REPRODUCTION PART III:
DEVELOPMENT AND FERTILITY

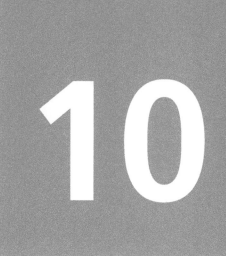

10

Chapter objectives

After studying this chapter you should be able to:

1. Explain the role of hormones in the control of sexual differentiation.

2. Explain the concepts of puberty and menarche.

3. Describe menopause and understand the use of hormone replacement therapy.

4. Understand the common disorders of sexual differentiation, delayed puberty and premature ovarian failure.

5. Understand how fertility may be regulated pharmacologically.

Introduction

Reproductive hormones are important for both sexes throughout life, starting with early fetal development where hormones have a key role in sexual differentiation. For teenagers, hormonal changes give rise to puberty. The previous chapters have dealt with the role of hormones in reproduction. This chapter covers the role of hormones in early life and up to puberty, then, in later life, the hormonal changes of menopause and the use of hormone replacement therapy. It also considers how hormonal treatments can be used to modify fertility, both as contraceptive agents and as therapies designed to increase fertility.

Gender determination and differentiation

There are normally 46 chromosomes in human cells: 22 pairs of chromosomes plus two sex chromosomes, either XX or XY, the female and male genotype, respectively. The presence of two X chromosomes in a fetus leads to the development of ovaries, whereas the presence of one X and one Y chromosome leads to the development of testes. There is a gene on the short arm of the Y chromosome, termed sex determining region Y (*SRY*), but referred to as the 'testis determining factor', that causes a testis to develop. The product of the *SRY* gene is a DNA binding protein that is able to modify gene transcription directly, initiating a cascade of gene activation which is required for the development of a functional testis.

Until 6–7 weeks' gestation, however, there is no visible difference between a male and a female embryo. At this stage of embryonic development, there is a primitive gonad which is found adjacent to two ducts, the Müllerian ducts and the Wolffian ducts (Fig. 10.1). These ducts will go on to form either the female reproductive tract (Müllerian ducts) or the male reproductive tract (Wolffian ducts). So at this stage, the fetus has the potential to develop both sets of genitalia. It is the fetal gonad that determines whether the fetus develops the male or female phenotype (appearance). The default option is female genital development, and this is what is seen if the fetus either has ovaries or does not have a functional gonad. This is because female genitalia develop even in the absence of hormone secretion by the female gonad: the Müllerian ducts persist and differentiate to form the fallopian tubes, the uterus and the upper part of the vagina; the Wolffian ducts simply regress.

Hormonal control of sexual differentiation

In order for male genitalia to develop, there must be an active over-ride of the default option. It is testosterone that functions as this over-ride mechanism, in conjunction with a hormone called anti-Müllerian hormone (AMH).

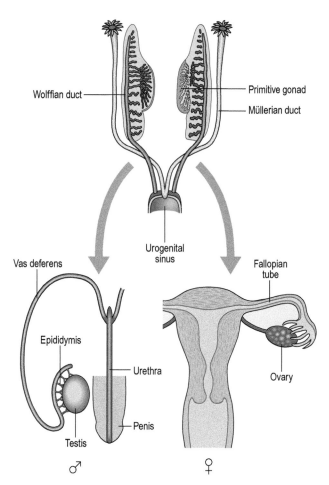

Figure 10.1 The fetal primitive gonad showing the arrangement of Wolffian and Müllerian ducts. In the male, the Müllerian ducts regress and the Wolffian ducts develop into the epididymis and vas deferens. In the female, the Wolffian ducts regress and the Müllerian ducts develop to form the fallopian tubes.

Case 10.1   Delayed puberty: 1

A 23-year-old woman presented because she had never had a period. In addition, her development had been behind her peers at school. She had been the shortest girl in her class and had never developed breasts.

The past medical history was unremarkable. She was taking no medications and was a non-smoker and took no alcohol. She lived with her parents. She had never had a sexual relationship or partner. Her performance at school had been poor and she worked as a sales assistant in a shop.

On examination, she was well, but shy and withdrawn. Her height was 149 cm (about 4 feet 11 inches) with a weight of 45 kg. She had short third and fourth metacarpal bones, a carrying angle at the elbow of about 15° and webbing of the neck. The skin showed a thick keloid scar over the site of a previous injury. Her sense of smell was normal.

How does an endocrinologist classify the causes of amenorrhoea?

Anti-Müllerian hormone is a peptide hormone closely related to inhibin and activin. It is secreted by the Sertoli cells in the testis of the male fetus and its secretion continues after birth until about the age of 10 years.

Testosterone is secreted by the fetal Leydig cells and is converted to 5α-dihydrotestosterone (DHT). The DHT acts to stabilize the Wolffian ducts, which can then develop into the epididymis, vas deferens and seminal vesicles of the male. DHT also acts to stimulate development of the male external genitalia. Meanwhile, the actions of AMH bring about regression of the Müllerian ducts.

These events all take place over a relatively short period of time quite early in gestation so that sexual differentiation of the fetus is essentially complete by 12 weeks' gestation.

Abnormalities of sexual differentiation

Abnormalities of sexual differentiation involving incorrect numbers of sex chromosomes are perhaps more common than you might think. Turner's syndrome is a condition in which a girl is born with only one X chromosome (denoted as 45 X O), instead of the usual two. Although there is only one X chromosome, the fetus develops a female appearance with female genitalia, because this is the 'default option' in the absence of a Y chromosome. It affects about 1 in 2000 newborn girls, although the great majority of fetuses with this abnormality do not survive past about week 28 of pregnancy. This is a serious condition which can include major abnormalities of the cardiovascular system as well as impaired ovarian function (Fig. 10.2). Women with Turner's syndrome are infertile and do not usually go through normal pubertal development and menarche without medical intervention.

Klinefelter's syndrome affects about 1 in 800 newborn boys. These boys are born with an additional X chromosome (denoted as 47XXY), although there are cases where there are multiple additional copies of the X chromosome. Although they are phenotypically male and appear normal as infants, there is impaired testicular function. As adults, males with Klinefelter's syndrome are infertile. They have small testes, which are often undescended, and there is a varying degree of androgen deficiency, which is normally treated with testosterone replacement therapy. We have already seen in Chapter 8 that Klinefelter's syndrome is the commonest cause of primary hypogonadism in men.

Thus it appears that the presence of a Y chromosome is sufficient to over-ride the default option during fetal development, but in the presence of more than one X chromosome, it is not sufficient for normal testicular function.

There are other conditions that can give rise to a range of abnormalities, from ambiguous genitalia to true hermaphroditism. If a female fetus is exposed to high levels

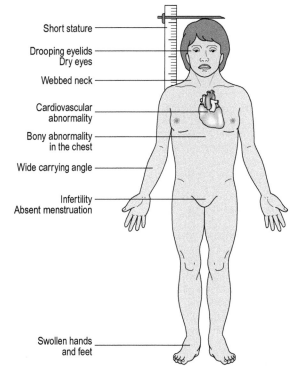

Figure 10.2 Features of Turner's syndrome (karyotype 45XO). In addition to the features shown, there is failure of normal pubertal development. The swelling of the hands and feet is due to lymphatic abnormalities.

of testosterone, particularly before week 12 of fetal development, this can result in the development of 'ambiguous genitalia', as seen in congenital adrenal hyperplasia (see Ch. 6). The androgens cause masculinization of the genitals, resulting in an enlarged clitoris and fusion of the labial folds.

There are two further genetic defects which occur in patients with a normal 46XY karyotype and which result in a female phenotype. Defects of the *SRY* gene have been reported in patients with a normal 46XY karyotype. This usually results in the formation of female external genitalia, but can present as a male phenotype with under-developed external genitalia. In both cases, there is significant abnormality of the gonads, with infertility and a greatly increased risk of gonadal tumour development. The treatment is therefore to remove the gonads and to give sex steroids appropriate to the phenotype at puberty. The second condition is a defect in the gene encoding the androgen receptor which results in androgen insensitivity (also known as androgen resistance). This affects around one in 20,000 people who are genetically male. The baby appears female but has no ovaries or uterus and is infertile. These people are usually raised as female and have female gender identity. However, they have underdeveloped testes located within the abdominal cavity, which may become cancerous if left in place.

Interesting fact

Some patients with Klinefelter's syndrome are chromosomal mosaics; in other words, their body cells are one of two different karyotypes (e.g. 46XY/47XXY). Chromosomal mosaics arise during cell division in a fertilized ovum and the result is a baby made up of two different cell lines. These cell lines can be randomly distributed in tissues (hence mosaic) or may result in some tissues being made up of normal cells and other tissues made of abnormal cells. In a Klinefelter mosaic, many of the gonadal cells will be abnormal (47XXY), resulting in low testosterone production.

Interesting fact

There has been concern over recent years about chemicals in the environment. Many industrial processes create chemicals with either oestrogen-like or anti-androgenic properties. There is, in addition, a considerable amount of oestrogen that ends up in river water downstream of sewage treatment plants. This comes from the urine of both normally cycling women and women taking the oral contraceptive pill. The effect of these chemicals in the environment has been to cause abnormal sexual differentiation in both fish and higher mammals. Male fish, living downstream of sewage treatment plants, have been found to develop an intersex gonad, containing both spermatogonia and eggs, although the eggs are not fertile. In the Arctic, there have also been reports of polar bears (who are at the top of the food chain and therefore likely to get a higher 'dose' of such chemicals) with both male and female sex organs: the true hermaphrodite state. The media has tagged the chemicals causing these effects 'gender benders'.

We do not know whether these agents also affect people. It is clear that there is an increased incidence of relatively minor developmental abnormalities in boys. These include cryptorchidism, where one or both testes have not descended into the scrotum, and hypospadias, where the urethral opening is halfway down the penis, instead of at the tip where it is usually found. There is also a well documented decrease in sperm quality in men living in developed countries over the past 50 years. However, it is not at all clear whether these effects can be explained by increased exposure to environmental chemicals, particularly given the huge changes in lifestyle and other environmental factors over this time period.

Hormones during development: puberty and menarche

It is not clear exactly what the hormonal signal is that triggers the start of puberty. There are various theories, but it is still not certain what removes the 'brake' on gonadotropin releasing hormone (GnRH) secretion by the hypothalamus. What is known is that the hypothalamus in pre-pubertal children is exceptionally sensitive to the negative feedback effect of the sex steroids, and the low steroid levels found in children are sufficient to inhibit the axis. There also appears to be a requirement

Case 10.1 Delayed puberty: 2

Amenorrhoea is defined as a lack of menstrual periods for 6 months or more. There are two major classifications. The first is between primary or secondary amenorrhoea. Primary amenorrhoea is when there has never been a menstrual period (as in this patient), while secondary amenorrhoea is a cessation of menstruation that has previously occurred. This classification is a clinical classification. It is useful in that a secondary amenorrhoea strongly indicates that the hypothalamo–pituitary–ovarian axis was once normal, suggesting an acquired pathology. By contrast a primary amenorrhoea is more in favour of a genetic or developmental failure of the axis.

The second classification is between a defect in the ovary versus a defect in the hypothalamus or pituitary. This is usually a biochemical classification, but can be suggested by clinical features.

List the biochemical tests that would distinguish between an ovarian disorder as opposed to a hypothalamic or pituitary disorder.

for the maturation of GnRH secretory mechanisms before puberty can occur.

As mentioned in previous chapters, the pituitary hormones luteinizing hormone (LH) and follicle stimulating hormone (FSH) are effectively stimulated only by pulses of GnRH. Although GnRH is secreted in a pulsatile manner throughout childhood, there is an increase in both the amplitude and the frequency of these pulses at puberty. It has been suggested that the pulse-generator in the brain is the key regulator of puberty. The net effect is that, with the removal of the hypersensitivity to feedback inhibition and the increased amplitude and frequency of GnRH pulses, LH and FSH secretion is increased, leading to greatly increased secretion of sex steroids by the gonads. This increase in oestrogen in girls and in testosterone in boys brings about the physical changes associated with puberty.

Pubertal development in boys

In boys, the first sign of puberty is an increase in the size of the testes which occurs as a result of increased FSH secretion, usually around the age of 10–12 years (Fig. 10.3). This is followed by an increase in size of the penis and a change in the colour and size of the scrotum, which continues until adult proportions are attained by the age of about 16 years. Pubic hair begins to appear during genital development after the enlargement of the testes. The growth spurt associated with puberty usually starts about 12 months after the first sign of puberty is noted and continues through the second half of pubertal development. The development of the genitalia occurs in parallel with development of pubic and axillary hair, and both are under the control of androgens.

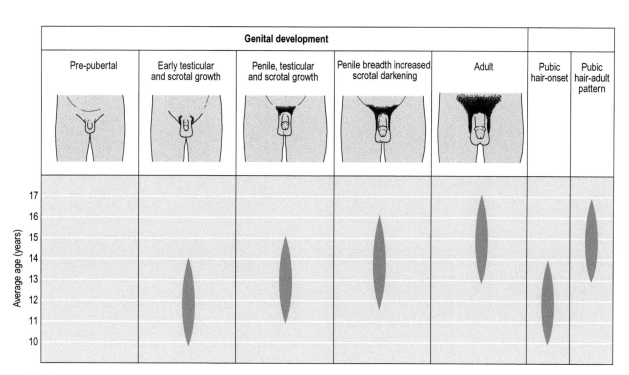

Figure 10.3 Stages of pubertal genital and pubic hair development in boys, with the average age of each stage shown.

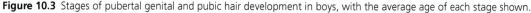

Pubertal development in girls

In girls, the onset of puberty is heralded by the beginning of breast development, which usually occurs from about the age of 10 years (Fig. 10.4). Pubic hair begins to develop at about the same time. Pubic hair development is usually complete by about the age of 15–16 years and breast development by the age of 16–17 years. The age of menarche (the first menstrual period) is determined by many factors including genetics, body weight, family size and season of the year (Fig. 10.5). Over the past century, there has been a progressive decline in the average age of menarche in the developed world. This has been suggested to result from a decreased incidence of childhood illness together with improved nutrition of children. The average age of menarche is currently about 13 years (with a normal range of 11–15 years), although there is some geographical variation.

Interesting fact

The decrease in the average age of menarche in the developed world since the mid-19th century, from 14–15 to 12–13 years, has been well documented. This has been attributed to improvements in diet and general health. However, what is not generally reported is that records from ancient Greece show that the average age of menarche at this time was 12–14 years. Similarly, in classical Indian civilizations (500 BC to 500 AD) the average age of menarche was 12–13 years, compared with 13–14 years in modern India. The implication is that early industrialization and urbanization is associated with a shift

to a later menarche, whereas later stages of economic development bring the age of menarche back down to pre-industrial levels.

Disorders of puberty

The onset of puberty can be delayed by several factors, including low body weight and excessive exercise, both of which are often features of anorexia nervosa. When

Case 10.1 Delayed puberty: 3

The simplest test is to check blood levels of luteinizing hormone (LH) and follicle-stimulating hormone (FSH). In this case the tests showed:

Serum LH	40 U/L (normal 2–10)
Serum FSH	60 U/L (normal 2–10)

Other helpful tests were:

Serum oestradiol	<60 pmol/L (normal 200–1400)
Prolactin	230 mU/L (normal <450)
Karyotype	46XO

Describe the significance of these findings.
What are the clinical risks she runs in the future?

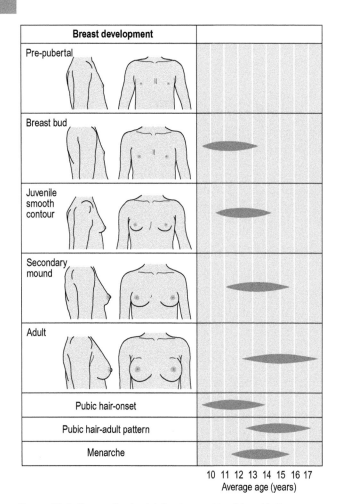

Figure 10.4 showing breast development stages:

Breast development	
Pre-pubertal	
Breast bud	
Juvenile smooth contour	
Secondary mound	
Adult	
Pubic hair-onset	
Pubic hair-adult pattern	
Menarche	

10 11 12 13 14 15 16 17
Average age (years)

Figure 10.4 Stages of pubertal development in girls, with the average age of each stage shown.

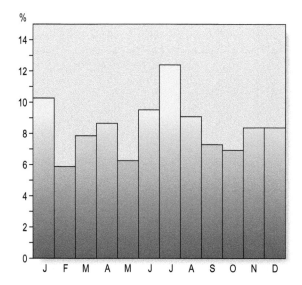

Figure 10.5 These data from the USA show that there is seasonal variation in the frequency of menarche. The graph shows the percentage of the study group of nearly 3000 girls recording menarche in each month. There were almost twice as many instances of menarche in July compared with February. The average should be about 8.3% if menarche is evenly distributed through the year. There was no relation found between birth month and month of menarche (data from Matchock R L, Susman E J, Brown F M. 2004. Seasonal rhythms of menarche in the United States: correlates to menarchial age, birth age, and birth month. Womens Health Issues 14:184–192).

anorexia nervosa is found in adult women, there is often a return to pre-pubertal patterns of gonadotropin secretion. Amenorrhoea (failure of menstruation) is common in these disorders, as we have already seen in Chapter 9. Overall, the commonest causes of delayed puberty are 'constitutional' (in other words, normal delay, which may run in families) and chronic illness (such as coeliac disease). There are additionally several much less common endocrine causes of delayed puberty such as androgen insensitivity syndrome and hypogonadotropic hypogonadism (see the case of John Smith in Chapter 8). As we have already seen, women with Turner's syndrome do not go through puberty without medical intervention and failure of normal pubertal development is often the reason why these women initially seek medical advice.

Delayed puberty is clinically significant. The epiphyses of the long bones fuse only under the influence of sex steroids produced during puberty, so a delay in puberty can result in excessive long bone growth. On the other hand, sex steroids are essential for effective mineralization of bones at puberty, and the absence of puberty can result in significant bone weakness. There are some very

unpleasant cases of bone fractures being seen in female gymnasts whose exercise regimes have had the effect of delaying puberty, thus causing weakness of bone structure.

It is less usual for early or 'precocious' puberty to be seen. In boys, precocious puberty is defined as pubertal development before the age of 9 years and requires investigation. In girls, early puberty is fairly common and tends to run in families. It is not usually due to an identifiable abnormality and, unless puberty occurs before the age of 6 years, would not normally be investigated. One cause of precocious puberty is congenital adrenal hyperplasia, in which excessive adrenal androgen secretion causes abnormal early genital development. This might be a good time to re-read the case history in Chapter 6 with the benefit of your increased knowledge of the reproductive system.

Gynaecomastia

When breast tissue is present in a man the condition is called gynaecomastia. It is a common condition, occurring in around 1% of men. The cause of this condition is usually an increase in the relative amount of oestrogen to which the breast tissue is exposed, although many cases are 'idiopathic' with no discernable cause. Normally, the high testosterone levels present in men inhibit breast development, but this inhibitory effect is removed if there

Case 10.1 Delayed puberty: 4

The investigations show ovarian failure, with an undetectable oestradiol level and high LH/FSH. The karyotype is abnormal, with only one X chromosome present. The patient has Turner's syndrome.

What are the clinical risks she runs in the future?

It is a feature of chromosomal disorders that they cause multiple other defects. Patients with Turner's syndrome suffer infertility, narrowing of the cardiac and aortic arteries, renal abnormalities, osteoporosis, autoimmune thyroid disease, autoimmune diabetes mellitus and relative growth hormone deficiency. There is no cure and medical treatment is mainly with oestradiol replacement to protect the bones from osteoporotic fracture. As Turner's syndrome is often diagnosed in the teenage years as a result of delayed puberty, oestradiol therapy is normally started on its own and in low doses. This is to allow the possibility of further growth as well as the development of secondary sexual characteristics, without causing fusion of the epiphyses in long bones. Sometimes, even though growth hormone levels are normal in Turner's syndrome, extra growth hormone is given to increase final height. After 1 or 2 years of low dose oestrogen therapy, the treatment is usually changed to the standard combined oestrogen-progesterone therapy (delivered paradoxically in the form of the oral contraceptive pill), cycling 21 days out of 28.

Case 10.2 Amenorrhoea: 1

Case history

Maria Lobo, a 32-year-old woman, attended for her annual review in an endocrine outpatient clinic 2 years after the successful treatment of her Graves' disease. She was worried that she may have a recurrence of her overactive thyroid gland because she had been experiencing increasingly frequent flushing and palpitations since before her last check-up. However, she also mentioned that her periods, which had become irregular 18 months ago, had stopped completely about 10 months ago. She had even bought a home pregnancy test, but this was negative.

Mrs Lobo had entered puberty and had her first menstrual period at the age of about 13 years. She had had two normal pregnancies with vaginal deliveries at the age of 23 and 26 years. She was taking no medication and used barrier methods of contraception. She exercised for about 60 min a week and ate a normal balanced diet. The family history was positive for autoimmune disease, with her mother and sister also having Graves' disease.

On examination, she was somewhat thin, with a weight of 56.3 kg and a body mass index of 20.6 kg/m². The thyroid was not enlarged. She was clinically euthyroid with a pulse of 75 bpm. Secondary sexual characteristics including breast and pubic hair development were normal. The remainder of the examination was normal.

What investigations should you request and why?

is either a significant increase in oestrogen formation or a decrease in testosterone production. There are several conditions associated with increased oestrogen formation in men. The commonest is obesity. Adipose tissue contains the enzyme aromatase which converts androgens to oestrogens resulting in the feminization seen in many obese men. Chronic liver disease and thyrotoxicosis are also causes of increased circulating oestrogens. Increased oestrogen may be secondary to an increase in human chorionic gonadotropin (hCG) secretion, which is a feature of some tumours. Decreased testosterone is seen in Kallman's and Klinefelter's syndromes, in testicular failure and in hyperprolactinaemia. There are also several drugs which inhibit testosterone synthesis including the diuretic spironolactone, the cardiac glycoside digoxin, and the antifungal ketoconazole, as well as the more obvious anti-androgens such as cyproterone acetate.

It can be very distressing for a man to develop breast tissue. In young men this can lead to social isolation with associated mental health problems. Although men can develop breast cancer, this is not usually as a consequence of gynaecomastia. If there is no obvious underlying cause then the only treatment is cosmetic surgery.

Menopause and the climacteric

Just as menarche marks the start of a woman's reproductive life, so menopause marks the end. After the menopause (the term applied to a woman's final menstrual period), normal pregnancy is not possible. Menopause is generally defined as the permanent cessation of menstruation as a result of the loss of ovarian follicles. It requires 12 months of amenorrhoea and can therefore be identified only with hindsight. Just as menarche is a single event within puberty, so menopause is a single event within the 'climacteric'. This is the term applied to the period of transition between premenopausal and postmenopausal states. In lay terms the climacteric is often referred to as 'the change'.

Until the 20th century, little was known about the menopause and the health of postmenopausal women, partly because relatively few women lived beyond their reproductive lifespan. It has also been suggested that the almost exclusively male doctors of the 19th century were more influenced by prevailing cultural stereotypes than by scientific evidence. Because menopause was seen as the end of a woman's 'useful' life, the menopause was associated with diagnoses such as 'feeble mindedness' and 'involutional melancholia' for which there was no evidence base.

It is perhaps surprising that, despite significant changes in life expectancy and a marked decrease in the age of menarche over the past century, there does not appear to have been any change at all in the average age at which women reach the menopause. The median age of menopause is 51 years and average life expectancy for women in the UK is currently about 80 years, giving a woman around 30 years of postmenopausal life.

Menopause occurs naturally as a result of the ovaries running out of follicles. The ovarian follicles degenerate and disappear, a process called atresia. It can therefore be seen as a physiological form of ovarian failure. This is usually not a condition of sudden onset. The ovaries become less sensitive to LH and FSH stimulation over a period of a few years with a gradual decline in oestrogen production. Premature ovarian failure can be medically induced as a consequence of either chemotherapy or radiotherapy. It may also be surgically induced by bilateral oophorectomy (removal of both ovaries).

Interesting fact

It is only women who experience the end of their reproductive lives so long before the end of their lifespan. It is thought that this reflects the fact that women are born with their total number of follicles, which cannot be increased. Men, on the other hand, have relatively unlimited capacity for spermatogenesis and usually continue to produce sperm throughout their lives, although there is a decrease in the quality of sperm produced by older men. Females of other species remain reproductively active for a greater proportion of their lives. Various theories have been proposed to explain this, but it may be a reflection of the length of time it takes for a human to reach sexual maturity and independence, compared with the young of other species.

Premature ovarian failure

This is defined as spontaneous ovarian failure occurring before the age of 40 years; it affects around 1% of women. Occasionally, there is an identifiable cause for premature ovarian failure, such as autoimmune destruction of the ovaries, but most cases are idiopathic. The reasons for premature menopause are not well understood but it seems likely that it may result from either a smaller than usual number of follicles formed during fetal development, or an increased rate of follicular loss after birth. It is not clear how either of these situations occurs. In both cases the number of follicles falls below a critical level at an earlier age than normal, resulting in primary ovarian failure.

Symptoms of the menopause

The acute symptoms of the menopause are usually attributed to the marked decline in circulating oestrogen seen during menopause. These symptoms can be divided into three groups: vasomotor, sexual and psychological

Case 10.2 Amenorrhoea: 2

Case note: Investigations
The following investigations were performed:

Pregnancy test	Result negative
Serum free T4	Normal
Serum TSH	Normal
Serum oestradiol	Low
Serum LH	Very high
Serum FSH	Very high
Autoantibody screen	Positive for thyroid peroxidase antibodies

All women of child-bearing age with amenorrhoea should first be assumed to be pregnant and a pregnancy test must be performed.

In view of her past history of Graves' disease, thyroid function should be checked even although Mrs Lobo is clinically euthyroid. Mrs Lobo has amenorrhoea, which could be due to primary ovarian failure or be secondary to reduced gonadotropin secretion. These can be distinguished by measuring oestradiol, LH and FSH levels. If the levels are all low, the cause is failure of gonadotropin secretion. However, Mrs Lobo's results show a low oestradiol concentration and very high levels of LH and FSH, indicating primary ovarian failure. Finally, the strong family history suggests that autoimmune diseases attacking the endocrine organs may be present in her and her family. Therefore, autoimmune disease of the ovary is a possible cause.

The presence of anti-thyroid peroxidase autoantibodies would fit with the idea that the ovarian failure is due to an autoimmune attack. Unfortunately, anti-ovarian autoantibodies cannot be measured reliably, and so cannot be used to confirm the diagnosis.
What is the diagnosis?

(Box 10.1). It is not clear whether the psychological symptoms, other than decreased libido, are the result of decreased circulating oestrogen, or whether they may reflect other life changes occurring at that time, such as children gaining independence, for example.

The major early symptoms of the menopause are hot flushes and night sweats. These are due to vasodilatation in the skin with a rise in skin temperature and sweating. The flushes are often felt in the upper body, head and neck, but also occur all over the body, and may be associated with palpitations. They may occur multiple times a day. Flushing occurs in any cause of hypogonadism where there has previously been some sex hormone exposure.

There are significant cultural differences in women's experience of the menopause. In Britain and the USA, approximately 70% of women report night sweating and hot flushes (called hot flashes in the USA). In other cultures, this percentage is lower. It has been suggested that diet and

Box 10.1 Acute symptoms of the menopause

- Vasomotor
  Hot flushes
  Night sweats
- Sexual
  Vaginal dryness leading to painful intercourse
  Increased incidence of urinary tract and vaginal infections
- Psychological
  Decreased libido (sex drive)
  Anxiety, labile mood.

lifestyle may be important in determining the severity of menopausal symptoms. The oriental diet, for example, is rich in soy, which contains plant oestrogens, believed by some to minimize the effects of the menopause.

There are, in addition, significant long-term consequences of the menopause. Osteoporosis is a major problem in postmenopausal women. Oestrogen deficiency results in a significant year-on-year decrease in bone mass, at a rate of about 1–2% of total bone mass each year. Although men also lose bone as they get older, it happens much faster in women, with the effect that about 1 in 3 older women has osteoporosis, compared with 1 in 12 men. Osteoporosis results in a significantly increased risk of fracture (see Ch. 12).

The effects of oestrogen deficiency on the urinary and genital tracts can result in vaginal prolapse and urinary incontinence. This, together with vaginal dryness, leads to an increased frequency of urinary tract infections.

It is generally considered that oestrogens are protective against heart disease. This is reflected in the lower incidence of myocardial infarction in women compared to men. The incidence of heart disease in women increases after the menopause, although the reason for this is unclear. Our current understanding is that hormone replacement therapy does not significantly alter the incidence of heart disease in post-menopausal women, suggesting that it is not simply a direct effect of oestrogens.

Hormone replacement therapy

It is clear that the menopause causes significant health problems in both the short and the long term. The use of hormone replacement therapy (HRT) to treat these problems is a controversial issue.

HRT is the term given to the use of oestrogens to treat menopausal symptoms. In a woman with an intact uterus, oestrogen administration causes an increased risk of uterine cancer. This risk can be reversed by the inclusion of progesterone in the HRT. So, for a woman with a uterus, 'combination HRT' is used, but oestrogen alone can be given following hysterectomy. A comparison of the dosage regimens typically used for HRT and the oral contraceptive pill is shown in Table 10.1 and the structures of the steroids used are shown in Figure 10.6.

Case 10.2 Amenorrhoea: 3

Case note: Diagnosis

Mrs Lobo had ovarian failure at the age of 32 years, and therefore had premature ovarian failure, which is defined as ovarian failure occurring spontaneously below the age of 40 years. The symptoms are the same as normal menopause. Iatrogenic premature ovarian failure may be a consequence of surgery, chemotherapy or radiotherapy. The causes of premature ovarian failure differ depending on the age of the patient. Genetic or chromosomal abnormalities usually result in failure of the ovary to develop and present with a lack of puberty and primary amenorrhoea (i.e. the patient has never had a menstrual period).

In Mrs Lobo, the ovaries had developed normally, she had had two successful pregnancies and there was a later destruction of the ovaries by the autoimmune disease process. Primary ovarian failure is part of the spectrum of organ-specific autoimmune diseases. In order to confirm the diagnosis, an ovarian biopsy could have been performed via a laparoscope inserted into the peritoneum and pelvis. However, this was considered invasive and Mrs Lobo preferred not to have this done.

By definition, Mrs Lobo was in the climacteric, with premature ovarian failure, perimenopausal symptoms and no periods for 10 months. By the time the investigations were completed and she attended her next appointment, she had not had a period for a year, so the end of her last period was retrospectively designated the start of her menopause.

Table 10.1 Comparison of typical formulations of the oral contraceptive pill, HRT and the morning-after pill

Preparation	Oestrogen	Progestin
Oral contraceptive	Ethinyloestradiol 35 μg	Norethisterone 500 μg or levonorgestrel 150 μg
HRT	Conjugated equine oestradiol 1 mg	Norethisterone 1 mg
Morning-after pill	None	Levonorgestrel 2 × 750 μg

Structures of the synthetic steroids are shown in Figure 10.6. Although a larger amount of oestrogen is used in HRT compared with that in the oral contraceptive pill, the conjugated oestrogen is much less potent than ethinyloestradiol.

HRT is very good at treating the early effects of the menopause, preventing both hot flushes and night sweats. Many women find that this also has a significant effect on their psychological symptoms, but it is not clear whether this is a direct effect or a secondary benefit from an improved quality of life resulting from better sleep. It is also clear that HRT improves sexual function, improving both vaginal lubrication and libido.

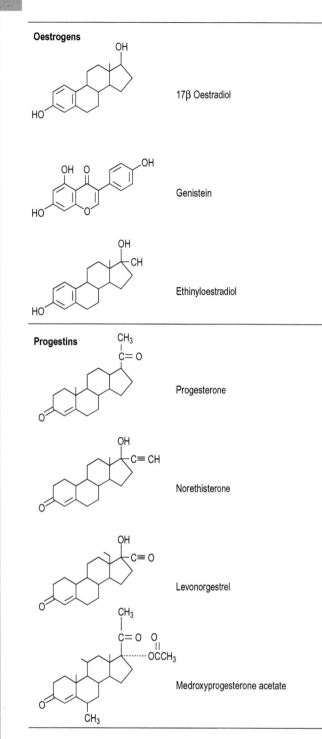

Oestrogens

17β Oestradiol

Genistein

Ethinyloestradiol

Progestins

Progesterone

Norethisterone

Levonorgestrel

Medroxyprogesterone acetate

Figure 10.6 Structures of steroids commonly used in contraception and HRT, together with genistein, a plant oestrogen. The only difference between 17β-oestradiol and ethinyloestradiol is the ethinyl group added at C17. However, this small structural change makes an enormous difference to the activity of the steroid; ethinyloestradiol does not bind significantly to sex hormone binding globulin (SHBG), unlike oestradiol, and undergoes very little first-pass metabolism in the liver. It is the most potent oestrogen currently available. Both norethisterone and levonorgestrel have the properties of a progestin, but structurally resemble a cross between progesterone and ethinyloestradiol.

Case 10.2 Amenorrhoea: 4

Case note: Future health risks

The main consequence of failure of ovarian hormone production is oestrogen deficiency, although the levels of other steroids, including some male sex steroids, also decline. The main effects of oestrogen deficiency are clinical symptoms and effects on bone mineralization. The lack of oestrogen results in loss of bone mineral, leading to osteoporosis and a risk of osteoporotic fractures. Dual-energy X-ray absorptiometry (DEXA) of bone mineral density is a useful guide to deciding whether osteoporosis is present.

The aims of treatment are to alleviate symptoms and prevent post-menopausal fractures. The main treatment used for Mrs Lobo was hormone replacement therapy with a combined oestrogen and progestogen preparation. Unfortunately, full HRT is associated with increased risks in patients above the age of 50 years (Box 10.2). The risk of endometrial cancer can be reduced by opposing oestrogens with progestogens. Bile cholesterol is increased in oestrogen-treated women and this worsens gallbladder disease. Some patients may still prefer full HRT if they have severe symptoms or advancing osteoporosis after the age of 50 years. A daily supplement of oral calcium should be added to Mrs Lobo's regimen. The bisphosphonates are effective at reduc-ing osteoclast action, improving bone density and reducing frac-tures. They should be used if there is osteoporosis.

HRT also has benefits for libido and vaginal secretion.

Long-term HRT

More controversial are the effects of HRT on the long-term consequences of the menopause. As with the drug treatment of any condition, there is a risk:benefit ratio to be considered. In the case of HRT the risks are still unclear. It has been hotly debated as to whether HRT causes an increased or decreased risk of cardiovascular disease. There have been large studies that have reported only marginal effects, so it seems likely that any risk, or indeed any benefit, is minimal.

One of the main reasons for long-term use of HRT is the prevention of osteoporosis. The rate of bone loss can be reduced significantly by taking HRT, and this is reflected in the lower rate of bone fracture in long-term HRT users. However, this protective effect lasts only as long as the HRT is taken. Once it is stopped, bone loss resumes at the same rate it would in the absence of HRT. It has been suggested that HRT may also prevent the development of neurodegenerative diseases such as Alzheimer's disease. However, despite several studies there is no reliable evidence to support this suggestion.

It is clear that taking HRT causes an increased risk of breast cancer and that this risk goes up further the longer that HRT is used. It is for this reason that many women choose to take HRT for 1 or 2 years, to treat the early

Box 10.2 Risks and benefits of long-term HRT use

Benefits
- Sexual health—HRT maintains vaginal structure and lubrication, and increases libido
- Bone health—HRT maintains bone mineral density and so reduces risk of osteoporosis
- HRT has also been suggested to improve cognitive function, wound healing and eye health
- HRT may also reduce the risk of cardiovascular disease, Alzheimer's disease and colonic cancer

Risks
- Breast cancer—HRT is associated with an increased risk of breast cancer
- Deep vein thrombosis—HRT causes a small increase in the risk of DVT
- Endometrial cancer—This risk is associated with oestrogen-only forms of HRT.

menopausal symptoms, and then move to alternative therapies to prevent osteoporosis.

Alternative therapies

There is a variety of alternatives to taking HRT for the long-term treatment of menopausal symptoms. Osteoporosis may be prevented by a diet rich in calcium and vitamin D, regular exercise and the use of bisphosphonates. These regimens have been shown to have as much effect as HRT in preventing postmenopausal bone loss and appear to have fewer side-effects.

Sexual dysfunction, such as vaginal dryness and discomfort, can be readily relieved by the use of a simple water-based lubricant jelly.

Some foods, including soy products, contain high levels of plant oestrogens (phyto-oestrogens) and various preparations of these are sold in health food shops. These are often marketed as 'alternative therapies' for menopausal symptoms, although there is no conclusive evidence that they work.

Interesting fact

According to the *Bible*, Abraham's wife, Sarah, was 90 years old when she became pregnant. This was, at the time, considered miraculous, but current records for the oldest woman to conceive are being broken every year as a result of advances in *in-vitro* fertilization (IVF) techniques. Proponents argue that it is a woman's right to conceive after normal menopause and point out that in previous centuries, when life expectancy was lower, it was usual for women to die before menopause. Opponents argue that there are good physical and psychological reasons why menopause occurs when it does and that pregnancy after this age is unnatural. What do you think?

Hormonal control of fertility: contraception

Oral contraceptive agents have a long history. In ancient Greece, both pomegranate seeds and pennyroyal plants were used as oral contraceptives. In the 7th century BC, a plant called silphium was in great demand as a result of its reputation as a highly effective contraceptive. It was exported from its native North Africa in such large quantities that by the 4th century AD it was extinct. We will never know what the active component of silphium might have been, but all the orally active contraceptive agents in use today are based on derivatives of steroid hormones.

During the middle part of the 20th century the great increase in our knowledge and understanding of the role of hormones in reproduction led directly to the development of hormonal methods of contraception. These fairly rapidly became the most popular method of contraception in the developed world. Until now, all hormonal methods of contraception have been designed for use by women. A 'male pill' has been undergoing development for at least three decades, but none is currently available.

The oral contraceptive pill

This is usually a combination of an oestrogen and a progestogen, although sometimes a 'progestogen-only' pill is used. The steroids are usually synthetic versions of the naturally occurring hormones; the synthetic oestrogen is usually ethinyloestradiol and there are various synthetic progestogens in use, including norethindrone (norethisterone) and levonorgestrel (Fig. 10.6). There are various combinations available and different schedules of administration, with perhaps the most common being the '21 days on, 7 days off' method.

The oral contraceptive pill works by mimicking the natural gonadal steroids and exerting feedback inhibition on the hypothalamo–pituitary–gonadal axis. This inhibits hypothalamic GnRH release and blocks pituitary LH and FSH release. In the absence of LH and FSH, there is no follicular development and so ovulation does not occur. The oral pill is also thought to cause thickening of the cervical mucus, presenting a physical barrier to sperm reaching the uterus.

The contraceptive pill is taken once daily. Its efficacy relies on efficient entero-hepatic recycling of steroids: steroids are conjugated in the liver and secreted in bile into the gastrointestinal tract, where they are de-conjugated and reabsorbed into the blood. This cycle is disrupted by certain antibiotics and by gastrointestinal disturbance, making the oral contraceptive pill much less effective at these times. Otherwise it is an extremely effective and reliable form of contraception, and is well tolerated by most women.

Long-term contraception

As an alternative to taking a daily 'pill', there are several long-acting hormonal contraceptive preparations

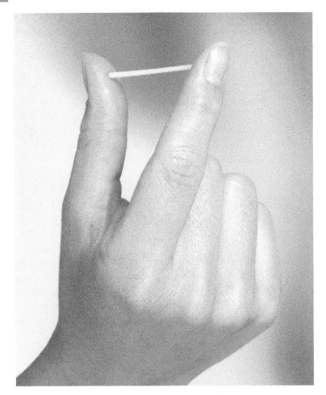

Figure 10.7 Contraceptive implant (courtesy of Organon).

available. There are two main forms of long-term contraception: the oily preparation of a progestogen, which is slowly hydrolysed, and the implant, which slowly releases progestogens (Fig. 10.7). These work on the same basis as the oral contraceptive pill but are administered much less frequently. The injectable forms last 3 months on average, whereas the implant lasts for up to a year. This form of contraceptive is not yet widely used, but the most common form of injectable contraceptive is Depo-Provera (medroxyprogesterone acetate). The efficacy of these preparations is not affected by stomach upsets or by other medication, and because there is no question of 'forgetting to take a pill' their efficacy is very nearly 100%. There are some side-effects, particularly 'breakthrough bleeding', although a new generation of combination implants has been developed to overcome this problem.

There are, in addition, a number of intrauterine contraceptive devices available whose efficacy has been improved by the inclusion of a hormonal implant.

Emergency hormonal contraception

While most hormonal contraceptives are designed to be used regularly in order to prevent pregnancy over a long period of time, hormones can also be used to decrease the chance of pregnancy occurring after unprotected intercourse.

The morning-after pill

A high dose of combined oestrogen and progestogen is used to prevent a pregnancy in the 72h after sexual intercourse has taken place. The effectiveness of this pill depends on how long after sexual intercourse it is taken. It is most effective within the first 24h. If taken up to 72h later, it prevents 75% of pregnancies, but it is much less effective after this time. The mechanism of action of this pill is not fully understood, but there is thought to be an alkalinization of the fluid within the uterus and a change in the structure of the endometrium, which together create an environment that is unfavourable for implantation.

Anti-progestogens

As pregnancy is dependent on fairly constant levels of circulating progesterone, one method of terminating an early pregnancy is the use of the anti-progesterone called RU486, or mifepristone. Mifepristone is a progesterone receptor antagonist, which prevents progesterone from binding to its receptor. It is effective both as a morning-after pill and for inducing termination of pregnancy at a later stage. It is an effective alternative to the surgical termination of pregnancy, which is the most commonly used method. The fact that mifepristone is not widely used is due more to political than to clinical considerations.

A male contraceptive pill?

There has been considerable progress towards developing a hormonal contraceptive for use by men. The approach has been to try to develop a regimen of hormone delivery that will inhibit hypothalamic GnRH release, as in the female contraceptive pill. Testosterone itself is the ideal candidate for this purpose, as it would allow potency and secondary sexual characteristics to be maintained. Supra-physiological doses of testosterone have an inhibitory effect on the hypothalamus and pituitary, shutting off androgen production in the testis and preventing sperm production. The main problem is that testosterone and other androgens cause liver damage when taken by mouth. To try to get round this, a testosterone skin patch has been developed. Most patches also contain a progestogen, as the combination of steroids is much more effective than testosterone alone. Several trials of these patches have been conducted but they are not yet available commercially.

Hormonal control of fertility: assisted conception

A woman who is not able to conceive naturally may undergo a number of investigations, including measurements of LH, FSH, prolactin, progesterone and testosterone. A woman who is not ovulating normally may be treated with a drug designed to stimulate ovulation.

Simple induction of ovulation

Clomiphene is an anti-oestrogen. It binds to oestrogen receptors and blocks the action of oestrogens in the circulation. It has been known since the early 1960s that clomiphene stimulates the release of gonadotropins and so can stimulate ovulation. Usually this treatment results in the production of only one or two eggs at a time, but occasionally can result in multiple births.

Preparation for IVF treatment or egg donation

Hormonal treatments can be used to make a woman produce multiple eggs in a single cycle. These eggs are then harvested and used for IVF. The treatment has three phases. The first drug used is buserelin, a GnRH agonist, which is delivered as a nasal spray. By providing the pituitary with a constant stimulation, instead of the usual pulsatile GnRH, gonadotropin secretion is turned off. After 2 weeks of this treatment, when the hypothalamo–pituitary–gonadal axis is thoroughly shut down, FSH is given by daily injection for about 10 days to stimulate egg development. At the end of the 10-day treatment, ovulation is induced with a single injection of chorionic gonadotropin (hCG) and the eggs are 'harvested' 36 hours later. Typically this treatment produces 6–12 eggs.

The harvested eggs are mixed with sperm and then implanted in the uterus about 36 hours after fertilization.

INSULIN AND THE REGULATION OF PLASMA GLUCOSE

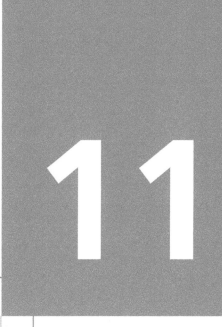

Chapter objectives

After studying this chapter you should be able to:

1. Explain how plasma glucose concentrations are maintained within a normal range.

2. Explain the mechanisms controlling the secretion of insulin.

3. Describe the actions of insulin.

4. Explain the consequences of a deficiency in insulin production or action.

5. Describe the main treatment options for type 1 and type 2 diabetes mellitus.

6. Describe the 'metabolic syndrome'.

Introduction

The brain uses glucose, its main energy source, at a much faster rate than any other tissue in the body (Fig. 11.1). It is perhaps surprising, therefore, that the brain does not keep significant stores of glucose. Instead, the brain relies on obtaining a constant supply of glucose from the blood. As a result, the brain is extremely sensitive to a fall in blood glucose levels. On the other hand, a sustained high level of blood glucose causes problems due to the increased osmolarity of blood; ultimately this leads to tissue damage as a result of inappropriate glycosylation in body tissues. Circulating concentrations of glucose are therefore maintained within relatively tight limits. This requires a complex system of control because plasma glucose levels can rise rapidly after a meal, but could also become very low during periods of fasting.

There are several hormones that act to increase circulating glucose concentrations, but the major hormone involved in lowering blood glucose load is insulin, a hormone secreted by the pancreas. A deficiency of either insulin production or effectiveness results in a condition known as *diabetes mellitus*. There are two principal forms of this disorder: type 1, which is insulin dependent (IDDM) and results from loss of insulin production; and type 2 or 'non-insulin-dependent' (NIDDM), which is a condition of insulin resistance (Table 11.1).

Interesting fact

The word 'insulin' comes from the Latin 'insula', meaning island, because insulin is produced by the islands of endocrine cells (islets of Langerhans) scattered throughout the pancreas.

Glucose in urine

Blood glucose levels are normally maintained at around 3–5 mmol/L in the fasting state. After a meal, this can rise to 7–8 mmol/L, but does not normally exceed about 10 mmol/L (Fig. 11.2). Above this level of blood glucose, the 'renal threshold' may be exceeded, with the result that glucose appears in the urine. Normally glucose, as a small molecule, passes through the kidney filtration mechanism into the urine and is then reabsorbed as the filtrate passes through the renal tubules. This mechanism involves active transport of glucose out of the urine and is facilitated by a glucose transporter, which works well at normal blood glucose concentrations, so that all the glucose is reabsorbed and none appears in the urine. At high blood glucose concentrations the transporter mechanism becomes saturated, with the result that not all of the glucose can be reabsorbed and glucose appears in the urine. This is called glycosuria, which can be detected easily and rapidly with a Multistick test. The presence of glucose in urine may suggest a problem with glycaemic control, such as diabetes mellitus.

The term 'renal threshold' refers to the minimum level of blood glucose that results in glycosuria. It is worth noting that the renal threshold varies greatly both between individuals and as a result of different conditions. For example, in pregnancy there is often a fall in renal threshold and glycosuria may be seen, without necessarily indicating a problem. Conversely, renal threshold increases with age and diabetes mellitus may not result in glycosuria in older people.

When glucose does appear in the urine, this causes an osmotic diuresis, resulting in increased thirst and urine production. However, in the normal state, the actions of insulin prevent blood sugar concentrations from exceeding the renal threshold.

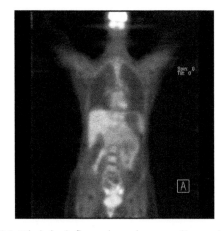

Figure 11.1 Whole-body fluoro-deoxyglucose positron emission tomography (FDG-PET) scan, showing sites of glucose uptake, obtained following administration of a derivative of glucose as a 'tracer'. The main 'hotspot' of glucose uptake is clearly the brain. Although it looks as though the bladder is also a hotspot, this is only because the tracer is being excreted in the urine (Courtesy of Dr Norbert Avril, Department of Nuclear Medicine, St Bartholomew's Hospital, London).

Table 11.1 Differences between insulin-dependent diabetes mellitus and non-insulin-dependent diabetes mellitus

	Type 1 (IDDM)	Type 2 (NIDDM)
Age at presentation (years)	<40	>40
Weight	Low/normal	Obese
Genetics	HLA linkage	Strong family history
Plasma insulin	Low	High
Ketoacidosis risk	High	Low

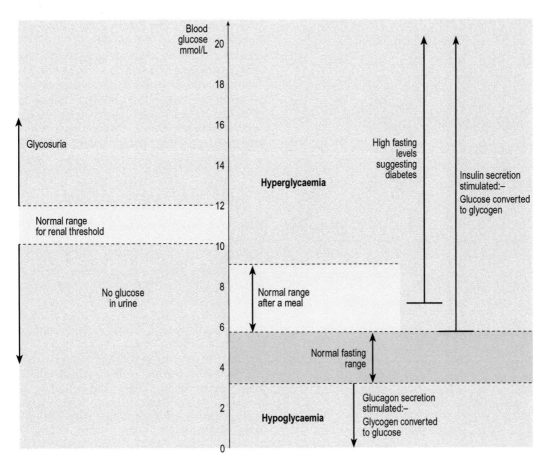

Figure 11.2 This diagram shows the normal range of fasting blood glucose and the normal levels after a meal. A fasting blood glucose above 7 mmol/L suggests diabetes mellitus. Glycosuria is seen when the blood glucose level exceeds the renal threshold, which is usually around 10–12 mmol/L, but is very variable. When the blood glucose concentration increases above the normal fasting range of 3–5 mmol/L, insulin secretion is stimulated, and levels below this range cause glucagon secretion to increase. These two hormones act to maintain blood glucose levels within the normal range.

Interesting fact

Diabetes mellitus (from the Greek for 'sweet urine') is so called because of the presence of sugar in the urine. In the days before the Multistick, the test for diabetes was to dip a finger in the patient's urine and taste whether or not it was sweet.

Insulin and the response to high blood glucose levels

Anatomy of the pancreas

The pancreas is an abdominal organ, with its head lying in the C-curve of the duodenum (Fig. 11.3). The pancreas is a lobed structure made up of the alveoli of secretory cells which drain into the large duct that runs the length of the pancreas and drains into the duodenum. The islets of Langerhans lie between the alveoli. The blood supply to the pancreas is from the splenic artery

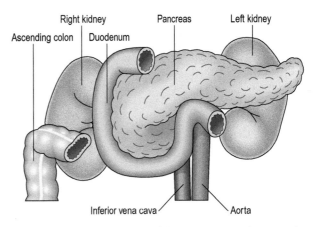

Figure 11.3 Anatomical location of the pancreas. Not shown are the liver and stomach; the pancreas lies behind these organs.

and the pancreato-duodenal artery, and venous drainage is into the portal vein. The pancreas develops from two buds off the duodenum, which migrate to join together.

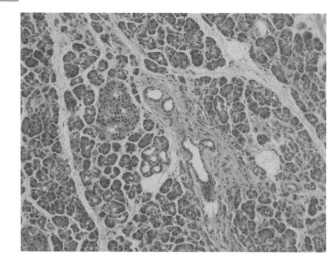

Figure 11.4 Histological appearance of the islet of Langerhans (courtesy of Dr Daniel Berney).

Table 11.2 Cell types in the islets of Langerhans

Cell type	Alternative name	Percentage of the islet	Hormone secreted
A cell	α cell	10	Glucagon
B cell	β cell	60–80	Insulin
D cell	δ cell	~5	Somatostatin
F cell	PP cell	Varies	Pancreatic polypeptide

The endocrine pancreas

The pancreas has two main functions: it produces digestive enzymes that are secreted directly into the duodenum (exocrine function); and it secretes hormones (endocrine function). The hormones are produced by the cells of the islets of Langerhans (Fig. 11.4), which make up only about 2% of the mass of the pancreas. Islets are composed of four main cell types which have two different naming systems, a Greek and a Roman lettering system. The commonest are the β cells (B cells), which secrete insulin, whereas α cells (A cells) produce glucagon, and the less numerous δ cells (D cells) and PP cells (also called F cells) secrete pancreatic polypeptide (Table 11.2).

In insulin-dependent (type 1) diabetes there is usually immune-mediated destruction of the islets of Langerhans, resulting in severely reduced insulin secretion.

Synthesis and secretion of insulin

Insulin is a two-chain polypeptide hormone which is made from a single large precursor called pre-proinsulin. This precursor is made in the rough endoplasmic reticulum of β cells where its pre-peptide is removed, and the

protein is folded and held in place with disulphide bridges between the A and B chains (Fig. 11.5). The resulting proinsulin is transported to the Golgi complex where the peptide is packaged into secretory vesicles for final processing and secretion. In order to make mature insulin, the link between the A and B chains is removed by proteolysis. This linking section is called C-peptide and is secreted with insulin into the circulation, when the secretory vesicles fuse with the plasma membrane in response to an appropriate signal.

Regulation of insulin secretion

The most important stimulus to insulin secretion is an increase in the plasma glucose concentration. This is detected by a glucose transporter protein called GLUT2 (pronounced 'gloot two'), located on the islet cells, in combination with glucokinase, which together are considered to be a glucose receptor. The GLUT2 allows entry of glucose into the β cell. The glucokinase converts glucose to glucose 6-phosphate, which is the starting point for glucose metabolism. The net result of glucose metabolism in β cells is an increase in intracellular ATP levels; this blocks ATP-sensitive potassium channels, resulting in depolarization of the cell and causing an influx of calcium through voltage-gated calcium channels. The increased intracellular calcium concentration activates calcium–calmodulin-dependent protein kinase, and leads to insulin secretion by exocytosis (Fig. 11.6).

Several other agents stimulate insulin release, including acetylcholine, bombesin, glucagon-like peptide 1 (GLP1), glucagon, cholecystokinin and glucose-dependent insulinotropic peptide (GIP), whereas adrenaline, galanin and somatostatin inhibit insulin release. Daily insulin secretion represents approximately 15% of the insulin stored in the pancreas at any time.

Insulin in blood

There is no specific carrier protein for insulin in plasma so it has a very short half-life of around 3–5 minutes. Insulin is metabolized by proteases in many tissues, principally the liver. The normal fasting insulin level is kept within a tight range and is dependent on the level of the fasting glucose. Usually for a fasting glucose level of about 5 mmol/L, the insulin ranges between 5 and 10 mU/L (35–70 pmol/L), with some variation depending on the insulin assay used.

What does insulin do?

Insulin is essential in the body as it allows cells to take up and then metabolize glucose. Without insulin the body cannot effectively handle a glucose load, such as a meal. In the absence of insulin, plasma glucose concentrations may be high but the cells of the body are effectively glucose deprived as the glucose cannot get into the cells.

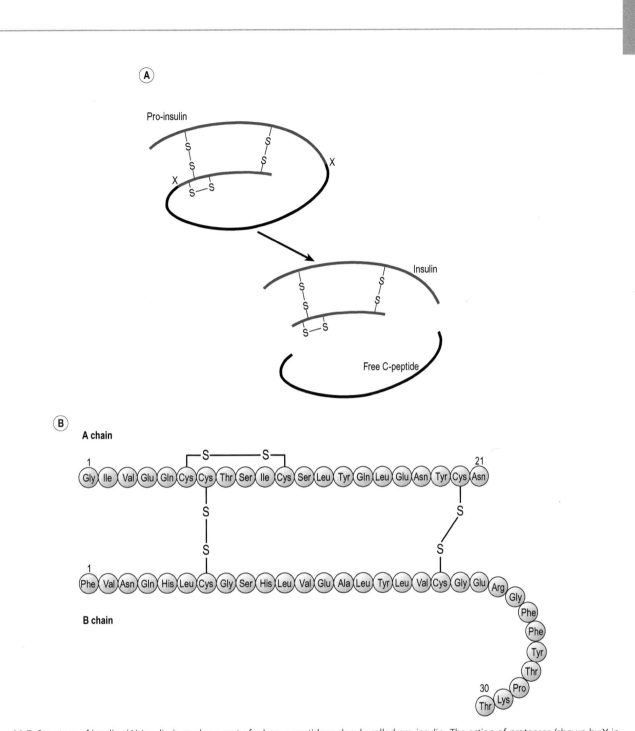

Figure 11.5 Structure of insulin. (A) Insulin is made as part of a larger peptide molecule called pro-insulin. The action of proteases (shown by X in the diagram) cleaves the pro-insulin to give the mature insulin and free C-peptide, or connecting peptide. S–S indicates the disulphide bridges that hold the two peptide chains of insulin together. (B) Peptide sequence of human insulin.

In most cells insulin exerts its effect by increasing the activity of a glucose transporter protein, GLUT4, at the plasma membrane, allowing effective uptake of glucose by the cell. In the liver, however, insulin does not affect GLUT4, but instead increases the expression of glucokinase, an enzyme that phosphorylates glucose prior to its conversion to glycogen.

The net effect of insulin action is to lower blood glucose by stimulating cells to take up glucose and convert it to glycogen. However, insulin has important effects on protein and fat metabolism in addition to its effects on glucose. Its overall effect is anabolic as insulin stimulates protein synthesis and lipogenesis. Insulin is essential in children for normal growth and failure of growth is one of the diagnostic signs of insulin insufficiency in children. The metabolic effects of insulin are summarized in Box 11.1. The glucose and insulin response to food intake is shown in Figure 11.7.

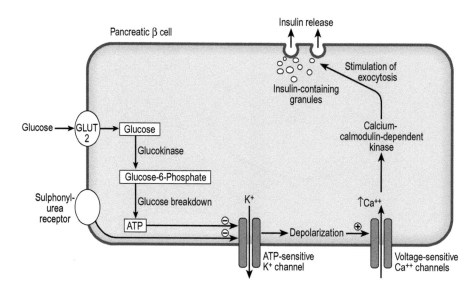

Figure 11.6 Mechanism of glucose-stimulated insulin secretion. Glucose enters the pancreatic β cell through the GLUT2 transporter. Inside the cell the glucose is converted to glucose 6-phosphate, then broken down to yield adenosine triphosphate (ATP). The ATP causes ATP-sensitive potassium channels to close, resulting in depolarization of the cell, which causes the voltage-sensitive calcium channels to open. The resulting increase in intracellular calcium concentration activates a calcium–calmodulin-dependent kinase, stimulating exocytosis of insulin-containing granules. This exocytosis is the mechanism by which insulin is released into the blood. One of the key treatments for type 2 diabetes mellitus is a class of drugs called sulphonylureas. These act directly on a sulphonylurea receptor on the β cell and have the same effect as an increased ATP concentration: closing the potassium channels and ultimately causing an increase in insulin release.

Box 11.1 Metabolic effects of insulin

Insulin is required to maintain all of these metabolic processes. In the absence of insulin these mechanisms effectively go into reverse, an effect that is further increased by the actions of glucagon.

Effects on glucose metabolism: promotes uptake and storage of glucose

- In muscle and adipose tissue—increases glucose uptake by cells, increases glycogen synthesis, inhibits glycogen breakdown
- In liver—increases glycogen synthesis both by stimulating glycogen formation and by inhibiting glycogen breakdown (glycogenolysis). Inhibits gluconeogenesis.

Effects on protein metabolism: promotes protein formation

- In muscle, adipose tissue, liver etc.—increases uptake of amino acids and promotes protein synthesis, inhibits protein degradation
- In liver—inhibits breakdown of amino acids to form glucose, decreases urea formation.

Effects on fat metabolism: promotes fat storage

- In adipose tissue—increases storage of triglycerides by inducing lipoprotein lipase and inhibiting intracellular lipase. Increases esterification and storage of fatty acids
- In liver—inhibits breakdown of fatty acids to ketones. Increases synthesis of triglycerides, cholesterol and very low-density lipoproteins.

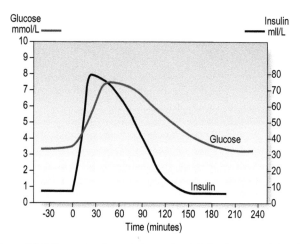

Figure 11.7 Plasma insulin and glucose levels following a meal. Levels of both glucose and insulin increase rapidly after a meal (time 0). The time taken for values to return to fasting levels depends on both the size and nutrient composition of the meal (from Chew S L, Leslie D. 2006. Clinical endocrinology and diabetes: an illustrated colour text. Churchill Livingstone, Edinburgh, with permission).

The insulin receptor

Insulin is a large peptide that cannot readily enter cells. It therefore exerts its effects by binding to a receptor in the plasma membrane of its target cells. The insulin receptor is one of the receptors which possess intrinsic protein tyrosine kinase activity (Ch. 2). It consists of four subunits and exists as a homodimer of one α and one β subunit (Fig. 11.8). It is interesting to note that the subunits of

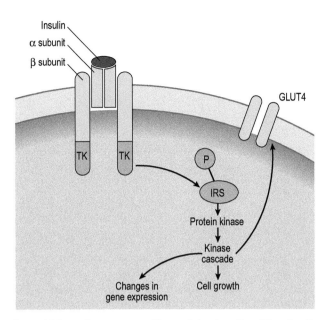

Figure 11.8 Insulin receptor and intracellular signalling. When insulin binds to the α-subunit of the receptor it causes the tyrosine kinase (TK) domain of the β-subunit to become active. This results in the phosphorylation (P) of intracellular proteins, and the activation of several kinase pathways, starting with the insulin receptor substrate (IRS) family. The actions of insulin lead to an increased number of GLUT4 glucose transport proteins at the cell membrane.

the insulin receptor are encoded by a single gene located on chromosome 19, which is expressed in nearly all tissues of the body except the brain, which is able to utilise glucose without the action of insulin. The receptor is synthesised as a single protein. The subunits are separated by proteolysis and then re-connected with disulphide bridges.

The α subunits are both extracellular and have insulin-binding regions. The β subunits have an extracellular domain which is attached to the α subunit, a transmembrane domain and, on the intracellular part of the receptor, a region of tyrosine kinase activity. An insulin molecule binds to the α subunits, causing the protein tyrosine kinase domains of the β subunits to become active (Fig. 11.8) and initiate a phosphorylation cascade, starting with insulin receptor substrate (IRS). One of the targets of IRS is the phosphoinositol 3-kinase (PI3K) pathway, which mediates the anabolic and growth-promoting actions of insulin. One of the main actions of insulin mediated by PI3K is an increase in the rate of transportation of GLUT4 receptors through the cell to the cell membrane. This has the effect of increasing the number of GLUT4 receptors at the cell surface, so acting to increase the capacity of the cell for the uptake of glucose.

After binding of insulin to its receptor, the hormone–receptor complex moves through the plasma membrane of the cell and collects in a specialized region of the cell membrane where groups of receptors are taken into the cell by the process of endocytosis. The receptors are processed in lysosomes where they are either degraded or recycled back to the cell membrane. It has been estimated that the half-life of an insulin receptor at the cell membrane is around seven hours.

In insulin resistance (see type 2 diabetes mellitus below) it appears that there is impaired signalling from the insulin receptor, rather than a defect in the receptor itself. Instead of tyrosine phosphorylation it appears that increased phosphorylation of serine residues on IRS diminishes its ability to signal through PI3K.

Glucagon and other hormones that act to raise blood glucose levels

Although insulin is the only hormone responsible for preventing blood glucose levels from rising too high, several hormones are involved in preventing blood glucose from falling too low. This 'multifactorial' regulation clearly reflects the importance of preventing blood glucose from becoming too low.

Classically, glucagon is the hormone that opposes the effects of insulin, and acts to raise blood glucose levels when they fall, thus maintaining blood glucose between meals and in the fasting state (Fig. 11.2). In reality, however, several hormones act together to respond to hypoglycaemia; the maintenance of fasting glucose is complex and also involves growth hormone (see Ch. 4), catecholamines and glucocorticoids (see Chs. 5 and 6). When there are disorders of these hormonal systems, such as excess growth hormone or cortisol secretion, hyperglycaemia and impaired glucose tolerance are often seen.

Glucagon is secreted by the α cells of the pancreatic islet as a 29-amino-acid peptide. Its release is inhibited by glucose and so it is secreted in response to low glucose levels in the α cells. The effects of glucagon are mainly on the liver, where it increases the rate of glycogen breakdown (glycogenolysis) and stimulates pathways of glucose formation from amino acids (gluconeogenesis). The net effect of these actions is to raise blood glucose levels. Glucagon also acts on adipose tissue to stimulate lipolysis, the breakdown of fat stores, producing increased plasma free fatty acid concentrations. In insulin deficiency (see below) the actions of glucagon contribute significantly to the hyperglycaemia and ketosis.

Disorders of blood glucose regulation: diabetes mellitus

Diabetes mellitus is the term used to describe the metabolic disorders whose common features are chronic hyperglycaemia with abnormal carbohydrate, fat and protein metabolism (Table 11.3). The cause is inadequate production of insulin, inadequate action of insulin, or both. By far the commonest type of diabetes mellitus is type 2 (non-insulin dependent: NIDDM), where the main abnormality is resistance to the action of insulin. The second commonest is type 1 (IDDM) where the main abnormality is insulin deficiency. There are some grey areas

Case 11.1 Type 1 diabetes mellitus: 1

Case history

Robert Smith was an 18-year-old student. He had arrived at his first term of university feeling tired. He initially attributed this to an increased consumption of alcohol in the first 2 weeks, but he still felt tired when he stopped drinking. The next symptom was passing a lot of urine. He needed to pass urine frequently in the day and six times during the night. The urine volume was always large. He also noticed increased thirst and would go to bed with a 1.5-litre bottle of soft drink to quench his thirst. He was regularly buying soft drinks during the day. He finally went to see the university health-centre doctor when he found his clothes were loose and realized he was losing weight. It was noted that his breath smelled ketotic, a characteristic sickly sweet smell that denotes an excess of ketones in the blood.

When Robert arrived at the university health-centre, a nurse asked him to pass a sample of urine for testing and took his weight (60 kg), height (1.75 m), pulse (90 b.p.m.) and blood pressure (115/75 mmHg). The following results were found:

Body mass index (BMI) = height in metres/(weight in kg^2)

= 19.6 m/kg^2 (normal range, 20–25 m/kg^2)

Urine dipstick testing: Glucose +++, ketones ++

After learning Robert's story and getting the test results, the doctor immediately told him that the diagnosis was insulin-dependent diabetes mellitus.

1. How does an understanding of glucose and insulin physiology allow the diagnosis to be made so rapidly?
2. Why did Robert lose weight despite eating normally?
3. How does an understanding of the action of insulin explain the ketosis and ketonuria?

Table 11.3 Causes of diabetes mellitus

Type	Percentage of cases	Cause
Type 1	10	Insulin deficiency
Type 2	85	Impaired insulin action
Specific causes	<5	Endocrine disorders (e.g. Cushing's, acromegaly)
		Pancreatic disorder (e.g. pancreatitis)
		Genetic disorders (e.g. maturity onset diabetes of the young)
		Drug-induced (e.g. glucocorticoid treatment)
		Part of an inherited disorder (e.g. Turner's, Klinefelter's)
Gestational diabetes	–	Insulin resistance seen in 5–10% of pregnancies

between the two types, with some people who have type 2 diabetes mellitus eventually becoming insulin deficient and needing insulin treatment but we will look at type 1 and type 2 separately. You will come across some of the rarer causes of diabetes mellitus, like Cushing's syndrome, acromegaly, glucocorticoid treatment, Turner's and Klinefelter's syndromes, elsewhere in this book.

Interesting fact

Diabetes was described in ancient Egyptian and Greek medical texts, but it was not until the end of the 19th century that the role of the pancreas was realized. Removal of the pancreas in dogs resulted in diabetes but, puzzlingly, injection of an extract of whole pancreas did not reverse the condition. We now know that this is because the insulin was broken down by proteolytic enzymes from the exocrine part of the pancreas.

It was Frederick Banting who in 1921 deduced that this problem might be overcome by ligating the blood supply to the pancreas in dogs, waiting for 6 weeks for the exocrine pancreas to die off, then producing an extract from the remaining pancreas. At the time, Banting's medical practice was not particularly successful so he took a job as a physiology demonstrator at the University of Ontario to pay the bills. He was unable to convince his head of department, John McLeod, of the value of the proposed experiment, but was eventually given a disused laboratory, a medical student (Charles Best) as an assistant, and 2 months to test his theory. The first ligatures were unsuccessful, but McLeod agreed to an extension of the project, which Banting sold his car to finance, and the rest is history.

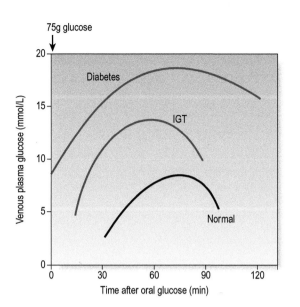

Figure 11.9 Normal and abnormal oral glucose tolerance test results. The figure also shows 'impaired glucose tolerance' (IGT) in a person who is developing diabetes.

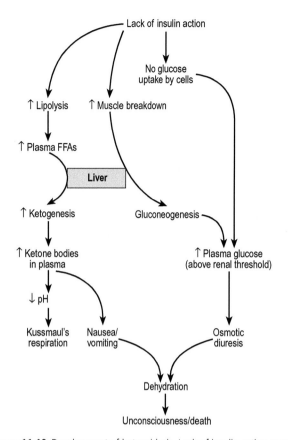

Figure 11.10 Development of ketoacidosis. Lack of insulin action means that cells cannot use the glucose in the blood, so need to get fuel from another source. The increased level of glucagon and other hormones stimulates muscle and fat breakdown, causing a rise in plasma free fatty acids (FFAs) and a further increase in blood glucose (from glucogenic amino acids). The use of fatty acids as fuel results in the production of ketone bodies in plasma. These have two effects: lowering of blood pH (the acidosis), and nausea and vomiting. The high blood glucose level exceeds the renal threshold and causes an osmotic diuresis. Together with the nausea and vomiting, this diuresis causes dehydration, which may be life-threatening. The acidosis results in Kussmaul's respiration: a deep sighing pattern of breathing in a physiological attempt to raise the blood pH by expiring as much carbon dioxide as possible.

The oral glucose tolerance test

An oral glucose tolerance test (Fig. 11.9) may be used to confirm a diagnosis of diabetes mellitus, although it is more usual simply to measure fasting blood glucose and free fatty acids. The test is based on measuring how the body deals with a glucose load. The person fasts overnight and in the morning is given a fixed dose of glucose, usually in the form of a sweet drink. Blood samples are taken at 30-minute intervals for 2 hours, and both glucose and insulin concentrations are measured.

Type 1 diabetes: insulin deficiency (insulin-dependent diabetes mellitus)

This is a disorder that is usually first seen in young people. The cause of insulin deficiency is the destruction of β cells in the pancreatic islets. By the time diabetes mellitus has developed, most patients will have no β cells left intact. This is probably the end result of a chain of events. There may be a genetic predisposition to type 1 diabetes, and there is some link to the human leucocyte antigen (HLA) genes. However, it is very likely that an environmental challenge (possibly viral) is needed. This leads to inflammation of the islets (called insulitis) and changes the nature of the β cell so that it becomes a target of attack by the immune system. Autoantibodies may be detected in the serum of patients with type 1 diabetes. These antibodies are targeted to antigens on the surface of β cells and are associated with β-cell destruction.

As a result of the lack of insulin, blood glucose levels are raised both after a meal and in the fasting state. As cells have a poor uptake of glucose in the absence of insulin, they cannot 'see' the glucose in the blood, and the body responds as if it was in a state of hypoglycaemia. Sometimes diabetes mellitus is referred to as 'starvation in the midst of plenty'. All of the regulatory mechanisms for correcting hypoglycaemia are activated, so there is increased lipolysis, resulting in an increase in plasma free fatty acids, with an increased production of ketone bodies, leading to the development of ketoacidosis (Figs 11.10, 11.11). This metabolic acidosis is partly compensated by a respiratory mechanism, called 'Kussmaul's respiration', in which there is an increased rate of deep breathing. This has the effect of causing greater total expiration of carbon dioxide, and so reduces the level of dissolved carbon dioxide in the blood, raising the pH of the blood.

In children, type 1 diabetes may present as failure of growth. The anabolic effects of insulin are essential for normal growth and development.

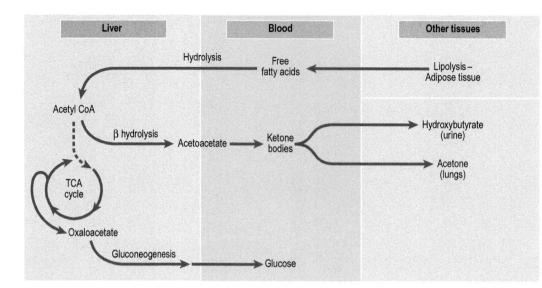

Figure 11.11 Pathways of ketone body formation in diabetes or starvation. Entry of acetyl CoA to the TCA cycle is impaired and so metabolism is diverted to acetoacetate and ketone body formation. Acetone is excreted via the lungs while hydroxybutyrate is excreted in urine. Oxaloacetate formed from the TCA cycle is diverted to a pathway of gluconeogenesis.

Case 11.1 Type 1 diabetes mellitus: 2

Case note: Diagnosis

The rapid diagnosis was based on the testing of the urine for glucose and ketones. Glucose is normally filtered through the glomerular membrane of the kidney and is nearly all reabsorbed at the proximal tubule. However, the capacity for resorption is limited. When high serum glucose levels exceed the capacity of the kidney (this varies but is at a concentration of approximately 10 mmol/L, or 180 mg/dL), glucose appears in the urine (glycosuria). This is easily detected by testing the urine with a dipstick. The detection of glycosuria by the nurse fitted with the finding of ketones in the urine and the clinical situation: young age, weight loss and symptoms of tiredness, passing a lot of urine (polyuria) and considerable thirst with high fluid intake (polydipsia). This led the doctor immediately to diagnose insulin-dependent diabetes mellitus.

The presence of glucose in the urine causes an osmotic diuresis. This is the reason for dehydration and thirst. Unfortunately, Robert's attempts to quench his thirst with soft drinks actually worsened the situation. This is because most soft drinks contain high levels of glucose.

Robert lost weight because glucagon and the other glucose-mobilizing hormones were responding to the lack of glucose available to cells by working to raise plasma glucose levels. These hormones act by increasing catabolism of lipids and proteins in the body, hence reducing body fat and protein stores and causing the weight loss.

Insulin is anabolic and produces polymers and macromolecules, such as glycogen and protein, from smaller molecules, such as glucose and amino acids (Box 11.1). It allows glucose to be used by the different cells in the body. If insulin is absent, cells cannot take up glucose efficiently, so the body 'looks for' another source of energy. In the absence of insulin, fat stores break down and release free fatty acids, which are in turn broken down into ketones. The combination of ketonuria and glycosuria strongly suggests insulin-dependent diabetes mellitus. The breakdown of glycogen to glucose, and of protein to amino acids, also contributes to weight loss and wasting of muscle.

Management of type 1 diabetes mellitus

Diet

A key aspect of the management of both type 1 and type 2 diabetes is diet and all newly diagnosed patients with diabetes should have a session with a specialist nurse or dietary advisor. It is important that dietary advice is realistic and tailored to the person's individual needs. It is not very helpful to simply give somebody a list of foods to avoid! The aim of dietary management is principally to avoid a rapid rise in circulating glucose levels. So the advice given is to avoid foods, like cake and biscuits, which contain simple carbohydrates (such as sucrose—normal 'sugar') and to replace these with 'healthier

Case 11.1 Type 1 diabetes mellitus: 3

Case note: Investigations

The doctor at the health-centre arranged for Robert's admission and treatment with insulin. The blood tests showed:

Plasma glucose	22 mmol/L (normal fasting, 3–6 mmol/L)
Plasma insulin	<5 mU/L (normal fasting, 5–10 mU/L)
Anti-pancreatic islet cell antibodies	220 kU/L (normal <60 kU/L)

How does an understanding of pathology and immunology explain these results?

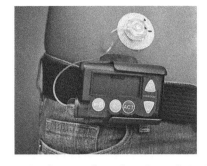

Figure 11.12 An insulin pump (from Chew S L, Leslie D. 2006. Clinical endocrinology and diabetes: an illustrated colour text. Churchill Livingstone, Edinburgh, with permission).

Case 11.1 Type 1 diabetes mellitus: 4

Case note: Explanation
How does an understanding of pathology and immunology explain these results?

The presence of high levels of anti-pancreatic islet cell antibodies shows that Robert's diabetes is associated with an immune-mediated destruction of the pancreatic islet cells, causing loss of insulin production. It is thought that an environmental event triggers the autoimmune attack in individuals with a genetic vulnerability. Certain genetic variants in the histocompatibility (HLA) loci on the short arm of chromosome 6 give a high risk of type 1 diabetes mellitus. The environmental triggers include infections (particularly enteroviruses). An immune response includes activated T lymphocytes and macrophages, which are found invading the pancreatic islets. Autoantibodies may become detectable in the serum well before the onset of clinical diabetes mellitus. These antibodies are targeted to antigens on islet cells, insulin, glutamate decarboxylase and insulinoma-related antigen 2. Islet cell antibodies predict a risk of future type 1 diabetes mellitus of 20–30%, compared with a general population risk of about 1 in 400 (0.25%).

options' such as fruit. It is important to eat small regular meals rather than one large meal each day as this gives a steadier release of glucose throughout the day.

Each meal should contain complex carbohydrates such as bread, rice, pasta or potatoes. Half of the daily energy intake should come from these foods. This produces a slow release of glucose from the digestive tract into the blood and can help avoid periods of excessively high blood glucose. Diabetes is associated with high serum lipid concentrations, which are linked to cardiovascular disease, so people with diabetes are also advised to avoid fatty foods. No more than 30% of the daily energy intake should come from fats, so patients are advised to eat chicken and fish which are lower in fats, rather than beef or pork, which have a high fat content. Patients are also advised to avoid fried foods and to replace dairy products with low-fat or olive oil-based alternatives. Vegetables are low in sugar and make excellent snack food. Fruit is also good, although fruit juice contains high levels of natural sugars which are absorbed much more rapidly than from whole fruits.

There is a range of foods made especially for diabetic patients. These often replace sugar with sorbitol, which is not absorbed by the gut and so can cause diarrhoea. In general it is better to save money by eating sensible amounts of normal food. One area where specific foods are useful is carbonated and other soft drinks, where the 'diet' version contains aspartame instead of sugar.

It is particularly sensible to avoid large amounts of alcohol if you have diabetes. Most alcoholic drinks contain high levels of sugar and low-alcohol beer and wine tend to contain higher levels of sugar than the full-strength alternatives. Alcohol itself has effects on glucose metabolism, initially causing a rise in blood glucose followed by a prolonged fall. This can cause serious hypoglycaemia overnight or at breakfast time following alcohol consumption in the evening.

Insulin therapy

For patients with type 1 diabetes, and also patients with type 2 diabetes who no longer have functional pancreatic β cells, treatment with insulin is required. Insulin is a large peptide hormone, so it is not orally active and must therefore be injected regularly. Various preparations are available, ranging from short acting to very long acting. Regular blood glucose monitoring is essential for people on insulin treatment. In patients given insulin for diabetic ketoacidosis, serum potassium levels fall quickly and serum potassium should be monitored and supplements given. This is because the action of insulin causes potassium to shift into cells with glucose. A relatively new development in insulin therapy is the use of insulin pumps, which deliver a continuous infusion of insulin subcutaneously (Fig. 11.12). These are particularly useful in people who find it difficult to achieve good control of blood glucose using other methods.

Measurement of blood glucose

At home

As the main aim in the management of diabetes mellitus is to enable the person to maintain normal blood glucose levels, it is important to have a simple method for measuring these levels that the patient can use at home and at work. Pocket-sized glucose monitors are widely available and give an accurate reading from a finger-prick blood sample (Fig. 11.13). People with type 1 diabetes are advised to check their blood glucose four to five times a day—more frequently if they are unwell or under stress. People with type 2 diabetes are generally advised to check less regularly as large fluctuations in blood glucose levels are less usual in type 2 diabetes.

Regular testing is generally thought to improve glycaemic control and lead to fewer long-term complications. This is partly because the patient can take appropriate action if the level is too low or too high, but also because monitoring glucose levels regularly allows the patient to learn the consequences of missing meals, eating cakes, etc.

In the diabetes clinic

Home blood glucose monitoring gives a useful 'snapshot' of the glucose concentration at that moment, but it is useful for a physician to get a picture of how well the patient is controlling their blood glucose over a longer period of time. The best measure of this is the glycated haemoglobin concentration (HbA_{1c}).

Haemoglobin in red blood cells naturally forms a complex with glucose. The amount of the complex formed is directly proportional to the concentration of glucose in the blood. Thus, measuring the proportion of haemoglobin that is glycated gives an indication of 'average' blood glucose levels. As red blood cells have a life of 120 days, the reading indicates how well blood glucose was controlled over the last couple of months. A high reading suggests that blood glucose has not been well controlled and the aim is to keep HbA_{1c} as close to the normal range (4.5–6.0%) as possible.

Complications of type 1 diabetes mellitus

Diabetic ketoacidosis

Hyperglycaemia may be the first presentation of diabetes, but in established diabetes can also be caused by an infection or other significant physical illness as well as by inadequate treatment. Because of the absence of insulin, the high blood sugar is associated with ketoacidosis and the dangerous resulting condition is called diabetic ketoacidosis. There is hyperglycaemia, with nausea and a characteristic sweet smell to the breath. See Figure 11.10 for an explanation of the development of ketoacidosis. Kussmaul's respiration is a deep sighing breathing that develops in an attempt to compensate for the

---

Case 11.1 | Type 1 diabetes mellitus: 5

Case note: Glycaemic control

Some 6 months later, Robert collapsed while out at a pub with friends. He was taken by ambulance to the Accident and Emergency department, where he was admitted to the hospital.

He recovered after treatment, but was very frightened by the experience.

Why did he collapse?

It is likely that Robert collapsed because he was not eating regularly. He would have been prescribed insulin in two forms: a long-acting and a short-acting form. The long-acting form is used to regulate blood glucose between meals, and the short-acting form is used at meal times. If somebody using the long-acting form does not eat regularly, they may become hypoglycaemic and collapse. The chances of this happening are increased by the consumption of alcohol.

Following his hospital admission, Robert was given an appointment in the diabetes clinic. A blood sample was taken and the results showed an HbA_{1c} measurement of 8.3% (normal range, 4.5–6.0%), indicating poor glycaemic control.

Robert was advised to monitor his blood glucose more frequently, and was referred to the diabetes nurse for advice on diet and lifestyle. He was warned of the consequences of poor long-term glycaemic control.

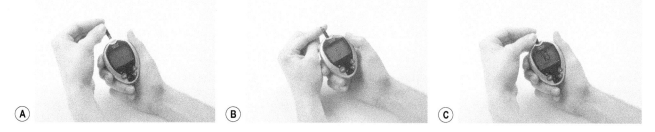

Figure 11.13 A home test meter for blood glucose level. (A) A new test strip is placed in the meter. (B) A drop of blood is applied to the strip. (C) After a few seconds, the blood glucose level appears on the meter screen. (OneTouch® Ultra® is a registered trademark of LifeScan Inc., image courtesy of LifeScan Inc.)

decreased pH. Deeper breathing decreases the partial pressure of carbon dioxide ($P\text{co}_2$), which causes a rise in pH. Ketoacidosis arises because, in the absence of cellular uptake of glucose, cells switch to metabolizing ketone bodies as a source of energy. Ketone bodies are formed by the metabolism of fatty acids (Fig. 11.11).

Hypoglycaemic coma

This is usually the result of taking insulin but not eating enough to maintain blood glucose levels. Blood sugar concentration is very low. This is a life-threatening condition that must be treated promptly. Many diabetics can tell when they are about to become hypoglycaemic and carry a sweet to eat in emergencies.

Type 2 diabetes (non-insulin-dependent diabetes)

In this disorder, there is usually normal or raised insulin secretion, but also a degree of insulin receptor insensitivity. This means that higher levels of insulin are required to achieve the same effect. It is therefore a disorder of *relative* insulin deficiency. Type 2 diabetes is far more common than type 1 diabetes, and is more likely to be seen in obese individuals. There are several factors that appear to contribute to the disorder, including a strong genetic

component, but the underlying mechanism leading to type 2 diabetes is not well understood. It is possible that type 2 diabetes is a group of closely related disorders, including the 'metabolic syndrome', that share the common feature of relative insulin deficiency (see below). The risk factors for developing type 2 diabetes are shown in Table 11.4. In the developed world the incidence of type 2 diabetes is increasing exactly in parallel with the increase in rates of obesity.

The result of the insulin resistance is that high levels of insulin secretion are required to maintain normal blood glucose levels. In many individuals this high rate

Table 11.4 Risk factors for developing type 2 diabetes

Age (over 40)

Ethnic group (Asian (esp. South Indian), Maori, Polynesian, black European/US populations have higher incidence than white European/US)

Family history

Western diet

Obesity

Physical inactivity

City-dwelling

Case 11.2 A case of type 2 diabetes with HONK: 1

Mrs Anne Baxter was an 84-year-old woman presenting with drowsiness and then weakness of the right arm and leg. She had been well until about 2 weeks earlier, when she had developed a chest infection. The first symptoms were cough, sore throat and fever. She became worse over the next days and stayed in bed. She refused meals and was taking liquids only, typically fizzy drinks. On the day of her admission, she became drowsy and did not respond to commands. Her husband also noticed that she was not using her right arm or leg.

The past history included a cholecystectomy (removal of the gall bladder). She was taking no medications, was a non-smoker and took one or two glasses of wine only once a week. Her mother and younger sister had suffered diabetes mellitus. Mrs Baxter was a retired cook and lived with her husband who was well.

On examination, she was unwell. Her weight was about 90 kg. Her temperature was 38°C, pulse 100 b.p.m. and regular, blood pressure 110/60 mmHg. She was dehydrated with sunken eyes and dry mouth. The chest examination showed dull percussion and increased breath sounds over the right lower lung. Mrs Baxter was incontinent. Her right arm and leg were weak and flaccid with mildly increased reflexes on the right side and an upgoing plantar response on the right.

Mrs Baxter was brought to the hospital by emergency ambulance. A finger prick sample was taken immediately on arrival and showed a capillary blood glucose of >33 mmol/L.

Investigations revealed the following:

Serum sodium	145 mmol/L (normal, 135–145)
Serum potassium	4.8 mmol/L (normal, 3.5–4.5)
Serum urea	21 mmol/L (normal, 3–7)
Serum glucose	48 mmol/L (normal fasting, <6.0)
Serum bicarbonate	20 mmol/L (normal, 20–30)
Chest X-ray	Right lower lobe pneumonia
Urine analysis	Glucose +++; negative for protein, blood and ketones
CT brain	Normal

1. Calculate the serum osmolality.
2. Characterize the clinical and biochemical abnormalities.
3. How would this help establish the likeliest diagnosis and the sequence of pathophysiology.
4. How does a knowledge of the pathophysiology guide treatment.

of secretion is not sustainable and β-cell function progressively declines, with some people ultimately requiring insulin treatment to maintain glycaemic control.

Management of type 2 diabetes

Type 2 diabetes may be managed by dietary control alone (see above), especially if there is a return to 'normal' weight. However, compliance with dietary advice is often poor.

There are two main groups of drugs used to treat type 2 diabetes: one group acts to increase the release of insulin from the pancreas and the other group acts to enhance the actions of insulin on target cells. The first group of drugs are called the sulphonylureas. They bind to specific receptors on β cells, causing the closure of potassium channels and resulting in depolarization of the cell, calcium entry and release of insulin (Fig. 11.6). It might seem obvious, but these drugs are effective only when pancreatic β cells are intact and functional.

The second group of drugs are the biguanides, the best known of which is metformin. These drugs do not require functional β cells in order to be effective. Their exact mechanism of action is not clear but they appear to exert several different effects, causing a decrease in hepatic gluconeogenesis, increased uptake of glucose by peripheral muscle cells and decreased intestinal glucose absorbance. Taken together, these actions result in a lowering of blood glucose concentrations.

As with type 1 diabetes, regular testing of blood glucose by finger-prick and periodic assessment of HbA_{1c} provides a useful guide to the management of type 2 diabetes mellitus.

> ### Interesting fact
>
> There is a new group of drugs which have been shown to be effective in the treatment of type 2 diabetes: the thiazolidinediones (TZDs, or glitazones). These drugs are synthetic ligands for the nuclear receptor called peroxisome-proliferator activated protein gamma (PPARγ). PPARγ is found mostly in adipocytes and has an important role in lipid and glucose homeostasis. Defects in PPARγ are associated with a particularly severe form of insulin resistance. Ligands for this receptor have emerged as potent insulin-sensitizing agents, acting to improve glycaemic control in patients with type 2 diabetes. These drugs do have adverse effects including oedema and weight gain, but research is going into developing selective PPARγ modulators, having the beneficial effects on increasing insulin sensitivity without the adverse effects.
>
> The Indian subcontinent has a very high incidence of type 2 diabetes, with an estimated prevalence of around one in six of the older population, and so affects around 40 million people in India. It has been known for many years that there is a strong genetic component to this disease in India. It is now thought that a defect in PPARγ accounts for a high proportion of type 2 diabetes in this population.

Case 11.2 A case of type 2 diabetes with HONK: 2

Calculate the serum osmolality (see Ch. 3, for how to do this)

- The calculated serum osmolality in Mrs AB is:
  $(145 \times 2) + 21 + 48 = 359 \, mOsm/L$.

Characterize the clinical and biochemical abnormalities

- This patient has a severe hyperglycaemia and hyperosmolality, but no evidence of an acidosis or ketosis. Clinically she has severe dehydration, a right lobar pneumonia, coma and a right hemiplegia.

How would this help establish the likeliest diagnosis and the sequence of pathophysiology?

- The diagnosis is hyper-osmolar non-ketotic coma (HONK).
- The first step in the development of HONK is a patient who is vulnerable to type 2 diabetes mellitus, but as yet undiagnosed. Next, an infection (in our patient, pneumonia) or medication (often glucocorticoids) causes a rise in blood glucose. The high blood glucose exceeds the renal excretion threshold. This leads to massive glycosuria and an osmotic diuresis (often causing incontinence of urine). This diuresis contributes to dehydration. The combination of dehydration and high glucose leads to an increased osmolality and thickness of blood. This, in turn, leads to poor blood flow, leading to cerebral symptoms,

such as coma and weakness in the right arm and leg. Ultimately, the thickness of the blood may cause multiple thrombotic events in the circulation. The mortality is usually >50% for each episode. There are several differences between HONK and diabetic ketoacidosis (usually seen in type 1 diabetes mellitus, Case 11.1: 1). However, the most important difference is that in HONK there is still sufficient endogenous insulin to prevent ketoacidosis, but not sufficient to control blood glucose.

How does a knowledge of the pathophysiology guide treatment?

- The main aims of treatment are:
  1. To replenish fluid losses with saline.
  2. Lower glucose with insulin treatment.
  3. Prevent thrombosis with low-molecular weight heparin.

In this case, Mrs Baxter suffered a cardiac arrest and died two hours after admission. The best chance of preventing her death would have been if she had presented to her GP soon after the onset of her chest infection. This would have allowed the GP to recognize her vulnerability to type 2 diabetes mellitus and to have checked her blood glucose. The main risk factors for development of type 2 diabetes mellitus are: family history of adult-onset diabetes mellitus and obesity.

Complications of type 2 diabetes mellitus

Hyperosmolar non-ketotic coma

As with type 1 diabetes mellitus, this is a hyperglycaemic state which can be the first presentation of type 2 diabetes mellitus or can be triggered by infection, serious illness or inadequate treatment. Because of the presence of insulin, blood sugar levels may be extremely high without production of ketones or development of ketoacidosis. It is still a very dangerous condition due to dehydration and the thickened blood being more likely to clot and cause blockages (stroke, heart attack and deep vein thrombosis).

Hypoglycaemia

In type 2 diabetes this is usually due to use of long-acting hypoglycaemic drugs and not eating, or taking an overdose. It takes a long time to correct this condition.

Long-term consequences of poor glycaemic control

The chronic complications of diabetes mellitus, regardless of the cause, are very clearly linked to the effectiveness of glycaemic control (Fig. 11.14). With good control of blood glucose these complications may be delayed indefinitely. Most of the complications arise from damage to small blood vessels. The effects of this include diabetic retinopathy and nephropathy, and may also result, in extreme cases, in gangrene.

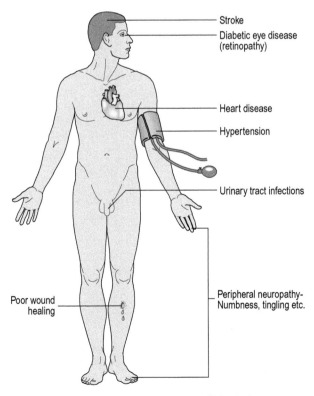

Figure 11.14 Complications of poor control of blood glucose in diabetes mellitus.

There are also effects on large blood vessels that appear to mirror an acceleration of atherosclerosis, causing increased incidence of myocardial infarction and stroke. In addition, poor glycaemic control is associated with a peripheral neuropathy particularly affecting sensory nerves, resulting in tingling, itching and other abnormal sensory perceptions.

There is also an increased incidence of infection and poor wound healing.

Gestational diabetes

A minority of women without previously diagnosed diabetes mellitus are found to have inappropriately high blood sugar levels during pregnancy. This is thought to be due to insulin resistance as a result of high levels of progesterone and cortisol during pregnancy. Although it is not usually symptomatic and blood sugar levels return to normal after delivery, women with gestational diabetes are at higher risk of developing type 2 diabetes mellitus later and their babies tend to have a higher birth weight.

The metabolic syndrome—a growing problem?

Most people in the developed world, if they have any interest in current affairs, will know of the serious concerns about the 'obesity epidemic' sweeping the USA and Europe. This concern is reflected in government advice on healthy eating, exercise and in the 'Healthy Schools' programme of the British Government in 2005. As a general rule, we are consuming more calories than we need and becoming seriously overweight. This is causing serious health problems in the populations of the richest countries, including an increase in a condition known as the 'metabolic syndrome'. This syndrome is a combination of common diseases that confer an increased risk of future vascular disease and type 2 diabetes mellitus. It has recently been estimated that 25% of all adult Americans have this syndrome. However, the metabolic syndrome is not simply a result of over-eating. It is also associated with other disorders, particularly schizophrenia, where there is a two-fold to four-fold increased risk of developing the metabolic syndrome compared with that in the general population.

Interesting fact

The metabolic syndrome is not a new concept. It can be recognized in classical clinical descriptions from the 19th century. For example, Samuel Gee, a physician at St Bartholomew's Hospital from 1866 to 1904, wrote:

'there is a diathesis which is very common, but for which it is difficult to find an appropriate name, because we do not understand its nature or essence. Among the diseases related to or dependent upon this diathesis are gout, gravel, obesity, diabetes, granular kidneys and arterio-capillary sclerosis'.

Diagnosis of the metabolic syndrome

The key components of the syndrome are central or abdominal obesity, insulin resistance, hypertension and dyslipidaemia (Fig. 11.15). A set of 'typical' blood test results is shown in Box 11.2. The clinical usefulness of defining a metabolic syndrome is still controversial and the condition has several other names (syndrome X, Reaven's syndrome or insulin resistance syndrome). A particular controversy is whether the combination of diseases carries a greater risk than the sum of the risks of the individual diseases. One major clinical benefit in considering the metabolic syndrome is that if one feature is found then the others should be sought.

Different criteria are used for its diagnosis, depending on the sponsoring organization. The criteria from the World Health Organization are shown in Box 11.3. The lack of a single consensus set of diagnostic criteria means that estimates of the prevalence of the metabolic syndrome vary, but most studies are in agreement that the prevalence in the developed world is increasing rapidly. Smoking has a further impact on increasing vascular disease but is not included in most diagnostic criteria.

The first description of the metabolic syndrome?

Samuel Gee described a case of a man in his 40s who was 'robust, even sporty' in his youth, but who has now gone to seed, drinking a bottle of claret a day, eating in expensive restaurants and smoking cigarettes. He has become obese with a flushed complexion, impaired glucose tolerance and hypertension. This cautionary tale concludes with the reprobate refusing to comply with his doctor's advice to change his lifestyle and, as a result, dying from a cerebral haemorrhage. (Adapted from Samuel Gee 1908 Medical lectures and aphorisms. Henry Frowde Hodder & Stoughton, London, Ch. 1.)

How is the metabolic syndrome treated?

We now know that the metabolic syndrome is not caused just by a surfeit of claret, and the clinical approach to the metabolic syndrome involves the aggressive treatment of each component. A diet and exercise programme benefits most patients, who should be advised to keep alcohol intake to a minimum. However, compliance with lifestyle

---

Box 11.2 Typical fasting blood tests in a patient with the metabolic syndrome

Glucose	6.8 mmol/L (normal 3–5 mmol/L)
Insulin	34 mU/L (normal <10 mU/L)
Total cholesterol	7.9 mmol/L (normal <5.0 mmol/L)
LDL-cholesterol	4.3 mmol/L (normal <3.0 mmol/L)
HDL-cholesterol	0.8 mmol/L (normal >1.15 mmol/L)
Triglycerides	5.1 mmol/L (normal <1.5 mmol/L)
Urine albumin: creatinine ratio	40 mg/g (normal <30 mg/g)

The key points here are: raised fasting glucose indicating insulin resistance; raised total cholesterol and low-density lipoprotein (LDL)-cholesterol with reduced high-density lipoprotein (HDL)-cholesterol, demonstrating dyslipidaemia; and a raised urine albumin : creatinine ratio, indicating early renal disease, probably as a result of hypertension.

Box 11.3 Diagnostic criteria for the metabolic syndrome as defined by the World Health Organization

Diabetes/impaired fasting glucose/impaired glucose tolerance/insulin resistance *and* at least two of the following criteria:

1. Waist:hip ratio >0.90 in men and >0.85 in women (central obesity).
2. Serum triglycerides >1.7 mmol/L or HDL-cholesterol <0.9 mmol/L in men and <1.0 mmol/L in women.
3. Blood pressure >140/90 mmHg.
4. Urinary albumin excretion rate >20 mg/min or albumin: creatinine ratio >30 mg/g.

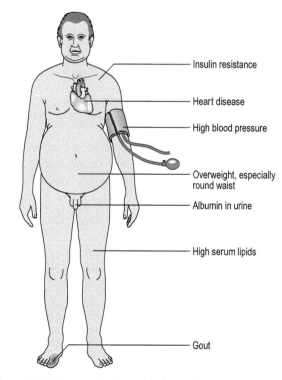

Insulin resistance

Heart disease

High blood pressure

Overweight, especially round waist

Albumin in urine

High serum lipids

Gout

Figure 11.15 Person with the metabolic syndrome.

changes is generally poor and most patients will require drugs to control lipid levels and blood pressure.

The lipids can be controlled with an HMG CoA (3-hydroxy-3-methylglutaryl coenzyme A) reductase inhibitor (a statin), which lowers low-density lipoprotein-cholesterol levels and raises high-density lipoprotein-cholesterol levels. The hypertension is usually treated with either an angiotensin converting enzyme (ACE) inhibitor or an angiotensin-2 receptor antagonist. This treatment both lowers blood pressure and reduces albuminuria.

There may be benefit in prescribing metformin (a drug that sensitizes the cells to insulin action) in addition to the other treatments. Metformin is a biguanide that has several effects on glucose metabolism. It reduces the production of glucose by the liver and increases the uptake and oxidation of glucose by skeletal muscle. There may also be a modest weight loss with metformin treatment. However, 'lifestyle counselling' remains the key to decreasing both the prevalence and the consequences of this very modern disease.

HORMONAL REGULATION OF PLASMA CALCIUM AND CALCIUM METABOLISM

12

Chapter objectives

After studying this chapter you should be able to:

1. Understand the significance of maintaining plasma calcium levels.

2. Understand the hormonal regulation of plasma calcium.

3. Appreciate the interactions between parathyroid hormone and vitamin D3.

4. Understand the regulation of parathyroid hormone secretion.

5. Appreciate the significance of renal function in calcium metabolism.

6. Have an understanding of disorders of calcium metabolism and metabolic bone disease.

Introduction

Calcium is a metal ion that is widespread in the body and has a wide range of functions. It is an important component of intracellular signalling pathways (see Ch. 2). It is also necessary for the activity of some enzymes and for the binding of hormones to receptors. An appropriate level of calcium is required for nerve transmission at the neuromuscular junction. However, most of the calcium within the body is stored in the skeleton, complexed with phosphate. The regulation of serum calcium levels is an important homeostatic mechanism, which is controlled by hormones, principally parathyroid hormone (PTH) and a metabolite of vitamin D3.

> ### Interesting fact
>
> Calcium accounts for 1.5–2% of adult body weight, so that the average person contains between 1 and 1.5 kg of elemental calcium, mostly in bone and teeth.

Serum calcium

Serum calcium concentrations are maintained within a very tight range. The normal serum calcium concentration is between 2.2 and 2.5 mmol/L. Approximately half of this is free, ionized calcium, and the remainder is either bound to plasma proteins or complexed, with citrate for example.

The consequences of plasma calcium straying outside these limits are significant. Hypocalcaemia results in hyperexcitability of the neuromuscular junction, leading to pins and needles, then tetany, paralysis and even

> ### Case 12.1 Primary hyperparathyroidism: 1
>
> #### Case history
>
> Joan Smith was 65 years old. She had become very tired over many months, if not years. The symptoms were so insidious in onset that she could not remember when they began with any precision. She had passed urine three or four times a night for several years. In the past year, she had become very constipated, passing hard stools only once or twice a week. In the last few weeks she had also been feeling nauseous.
>
> The past history included an episode of renal colic about 15 years previously. Mrs Smith had passed the stone in her urine.
>
> On examination, she appeared fatigued and low in mood. Her blood pressure was 165/95 mmHg. There were several mobile lumps in the abdomen which were thought to be hard faeces in the colon. The rectum contained hard faeces.

convulsions, whereas chronic hypercalcaemia may result in the formation of kidney stones (renal calculi), constipation, dehydration, kidney damage, tiredness and depression.

> ### Interesting fact
>
> It is the free, ionized calcium in plasma that is physiologically active, but common laboratory tests measure total calcium, which includes that which is bound to albumin and other proteins. Increases or decreases in the levels of these plasma proteins will obviously affect the amounts of physiologically active calcium in the blood, so the total calcium is 'corrected' to take account of the albumin concentration. It is this corrected value that is used to determine whether the calcium levels are abnormal.

Sources of serum calcium

The vast bulk of the body's calcium store is stored in the skeleton. Although the skeleton is often considered to be simply structural, bone is a readily available source of calcium and will be sacrificed if necessary to maintain serum calcium levels (Fig. 12.1). Calcium is also actively reabsorbed in the kidney and dietary calcium is absorbed from the gut. This latter source is the only mechanism by which total body calcium can be increased, so it is important that this absorption occurs efficiently, especially in children and pregnant women who need to be in positive calcium balance. The availability of calcium from each of these sources is under hormonal control.

In order to understand the regulation of plasma calcium it is really necessary to have a look at the physiology of bone.

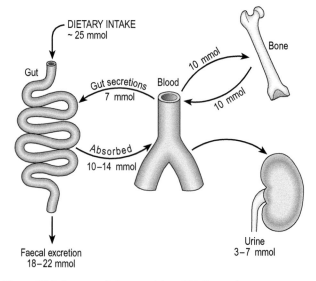

Figure 12.1 Sources of plasma calcium. This figure shows approximate daily calcium turnover for an adult in calcium balance. It is important to recognize that calcium in bone is not all fixed, but can contribute to plasma levels of calcium.

The structure, functions and endocrinology of bone

Bone, as well as providing a rigid protective support for the body and a site of attachment for muscles, also provides a large reservoir of minerals, especially calcium and phosphate, for the body. The hollow core of bone contains the bone marrow which is the main site of production of new blood cells.

Bone is made up of a basic extracellular collagen matrix, which is heavily mineralized with calcium and phosphate salts, surrounding a loose network of cells called osteocytes (Fig. 12.2). The major mineral in bone is called hydroxyapatite and is a crystalline complex of calcium and phosphate. The skeleton may appear to be a solid unchanging structure, but the key to understanding calcium metabolism and bone physiology is the fact that bone is constantly changing, being broken down and built up again. These processes are termed bone resorption and bone formation and it is the balance between them that is important. In healthy adults the rate of bone resorption is usually equal to the rate of formation, but under some circumstances there is a greater rate of resorption which can lead to bone disease. It has been estimated that 20% of all the calcium in bone turns over each year in an adult. This rate of turnover is far higher in children.

Bone growth

During development, the long bones form initially as cartilage which is transformed into bone by a process called ossification. Throughout childhood the long bones grow in length through a process involving cartilage formation and ossification. If this were to occur at the ends of the bone it would cause functional joint problems so instead the growth mainly occurs between the shaft of the bone and the joint, at sites called the epiphyses (Fig. 12.2). Long bone growth only continues for as long as the epiphyses remain functional. At puberty, under the influence of the sex steroids, testosterone and oestradiol, the cartilage cells stop dividing, become ossified and fuse with the shaft of the bone. This process is termed epiphyseal closure and means that further growth of the long bone is not possible.

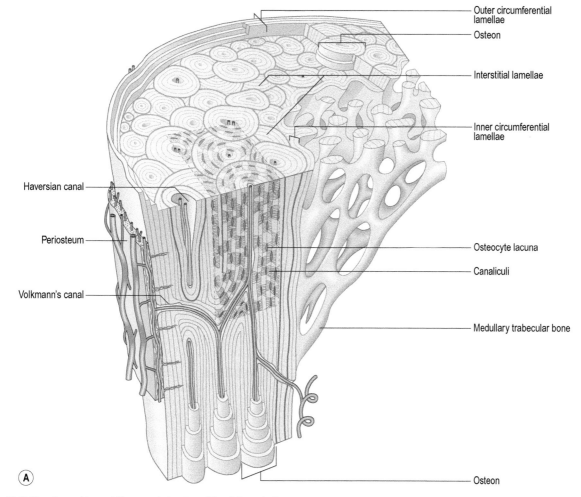

Figure 12.2 Structure of bone (A) general structure (B) epiphyseal plate.

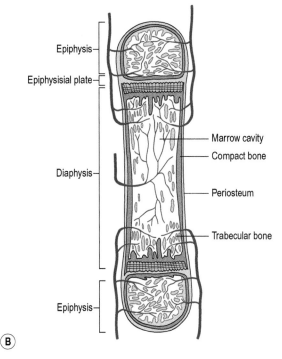

Figure 12.2 (Continued).

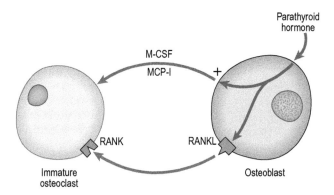

Figure 12.3 Communication between osteoclasts and osteoblasts. Osteoblasts produce RANKL, which binds to the RANK receptor on immature osteoclasts. RANKL is expressed on the cell surface of osteoblasts and so the cells need to be in direct contact for receptor activation to occur. Osteoblasts also secrete M-CSF (monocyte colony stimulating factor) and MCP-1 (monocyte chemoattractant protein) which both bind to immature osteoclasts and have a role in osteoclast recruitment and maturation. The expression of these factors by osteoblasts is stimulated by parathyroid hormone. A wide range of other factors is also produced by both osteoclasts and osteoblasts, so there is two-way communication between these cell types.

Bone cells

There are several cell types which make up the structure of bone. The cells responsible for bone formation are the osteoblasts. These are modified fibroblasts and function to make new collagen and create the right microclimate for mineralization of bone. The cells responsible for bone resorption are called osteoclasts, and are differentiated monocytes, large multinucleated cells produced in the bone marrow. Osteoclasts act to reabsorb bone by attaching to the bone and using proton pumps to acidify the area of bone beneath the osteoclast. The acid dissolves the hydroxyapatite crystals and the osteoclast secretes an enzyme called an acid protease to break down the collagen. The osteoclast absorbs both the mineral and the protein and releases them into intercellular fluid. Once the osteoclast has dissolved a pit in the bone, the osteoblasts move in and begin the process of making bone collagen, osteoid. As the osteoid forms and attracts hydroxyapatite crystals, the osteoblasts become trapped and transform into osteocytes, which connect with other osteocytes through the bone. Their function is not fully understood but it appears that they may have a role in sensing mechanical stress on the bone.

These cells are not randomly distributed but are organized into bone remodelling units with several osteoblasts associated with each osteoclast. It has been calculated that there are two million remodelling units working in each person at any given time. The two cell types are so closely associated that it is not surprising to learn that

there is active communication between them. The osteoblasts produce an osteoclast activating factor: RANKL (receptor activator of NF-KB ligand) which binds to the RANK receptor on osteoclasts (Fig. 12.3). Production of RANKL is under the direct control of parathyroid hormone. Other aspects of osteoclast and osteoblast function are also under endocrine control.

Case 12.1	Primary hyperparathyroidism: 2

Case note: Investigations

Mrs Smith has a history and symptoms that suggest chronic hypercalcaemia. Investigations were requested, including blood tests, abdominal radiography, and a urine specimen for microbiology and cytology.

The endocrinology of bone

The hormonal regulation of bone is effected mainly through the actions of two hormones: parathyroid hormone and calcitriol (see below for details of their actions). PTH is the major regulator: its receptors are expressed on osteoblasts but not on osteoclasts. It stimulates osteoblast activity and, in particular, cell survival. However, high levels of PTH for a longer period of time cause a shift in the balance of cell activity, favouring osteoclast activity and bone resorption. PTH achieves this by stimulating the osteoblasts to secrete an osteoclast stimulating factor: RANKL, rather than acting directly on osteoclast cells. Calcitriol, which is a metabolite of vitamin D, appears to have a permissive effect on osteoblast function that is not well-understood.

Growth hormone is the most significant stimulus for bone growth during childhood. These effects are at least partly mediated by locally produced IGF-1 which stimulates proliferation of cartilage cells in the epiphyseal plate, and has local metabolic effects which favour bone formation (see Ch. 4).

Sex steroids have important effects on bone: oestrogens promote osteoblast function and stimulate apoptosis of osteoclasts and so promote bone formation. Oestrogens also promote calcium uptake in the gut. Androgens are also anabolic in bone but exert most of these effects after local conversion to oestrogens. Glucocorticoids, in contrast, are catabolic in bone, promoting osteoclast activity and also inhibiting calcium uptake in the gut. Osteoporosis is a significant adverse effect of long-term treatment with glucocorticoid therapy (see Ch. 6).

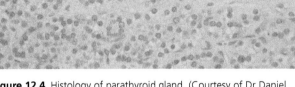

Figure 12.4 Histology of parathyroid gland. (Courtesy of Dr Daniel Berney.)

Interesting fact

You can easily remember the difference between osteoblasts and osteoclasts because 'Blasts are Builders', whereas 'Clasts Claw away bone'.

Hormones involved in the regulation of serum calcium

Given the consequences of dysregulation of serum calcium, it is clearly important that levels are maintained within set limits. The two key hormones involved in the regulation of serum calcium concentrations: PTH and calcitriol both raise serum calcium concentrations, but act by different mechanisms and over quite different timescales. The short-term regulation of serum calcium is under the control of PTH, whereas calcitriol is responsible for longer-term regulation.

Parathyroid hormone

The parathyroid glands

PTH is secreted by the chief cells of the parathyroid gland (Fig. 12.4). There are usually four parathyroid glands, located on the posterior surface of the thyroid gland. These glands are small in size, each weighing around 50 mg, but may weigh as much as 70 mg. Women usually have larger parathyroid glands than men. Embryologically, the superior and inferior pairs of parathyroid glands have different origins, although both are endodermal. The superior pair of parathyroids derive from the fourth branchial pouch and do not migrate during fetal development, while the inferior parathyroids develop from the third branchial pouch and migrate caudally to sit at the lower pole of the thyroid gland. Changes in this migratory process appear to account for the rather variable position of the lower parathyroid glands.

Interesting fact

Although there are usually four parathyroid glands, there is a great variation between individuals. One person was reported to have 104 distinct parathyroid glands, located throughout the neck region. The parathyroids are usually found attached to the thyroid gland, but may be found in other locations, including being embedded within the thyroid itself, or attached to the oesophagus.

Secretion of parathyroid hormone

PTH is a peptide hormone comprising 84 amino acids, encoded by a gene on chromosome 11. It is synthesized as a larger precursor, termed preproPTH and processed to the final secreted form as it moves through the cell from the endoplasmic reticulum and Golgi body, with the final processing taking place in the secretory vesicle. The preproPTH has 29 amino acids removed in the endoplasmic reticulum to yield pro-PTH. This is translocated to the Golgi, and six further residues are removed, by the action of a peptidase, to yield the final mature PTH. Like most peptide hormones, it is stored in secretory vesicles within the cells and rapidly released when required. Unusually for peptide hormones, the pro-PTH form is not secreted in any significant amount.

Secretion of PTH is stimulated mainly by a low serum calcium concentration and inhibited by high serum calcium (Fig. 12.5). There are specific calcium-sensing receptors (CaR) on the surface of the chief cells that monitor serum calcium levels. These receptors are so sensitive

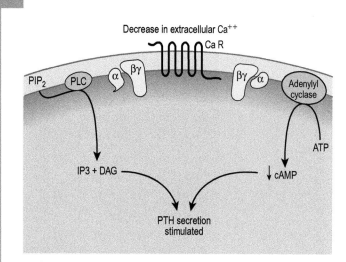

Figure 12.5 Regulation of parathyroid hormone (PTH) secretion. This is a very simple regulatory system. Calcium-sensitive receptors on the secretory cells respond to changes in plasma calcium concentrations; a low plasma calcium level stimulates PTH secretion while a high concentration is inhibitory. Plasma calcium is detected by a G-protein coupled calcium receptor (CaR). Two second messenger systems mediate these effects: AC adenylyl cyclase, PLC phospholipase C. Activation of the CaR causes stimulation of PLC and inhibition of AC.

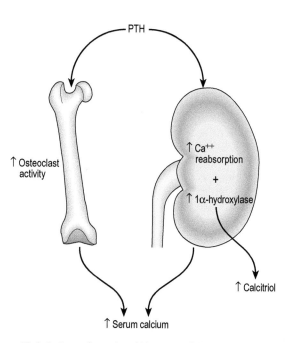

Figure 12.6 Actions of parathyroid hormone (PTH). The target organs are bone and kidney. PTH has a rapid effect on these tissues, stimulating calcium resorption from urine and activating osteoclasts. PTH also stimulates the activation of vitamin D in the kidney.

to changes in serum calcium that a fall of as little as 0.1 mmol/L is sufficient to cause maximal secretion of PTH. The CaR is a member of the same family of G-protein coupled receptors as smell and taste receptors. It is coupled to inhibition of adenylyl cyclase and activation of phospholipase C and MAP kinase pathways (see Ch. 2). CaR is also expressed in the kidney, bone and the gastrointestinal system and is thought to have a role in coordinating the body's calcium homeostatic mechanisms. Mutations in the CaR may be activating or inactivating. Activating mutations result in a low plasma calcium because the parathyroid gland is over-sensitive to plasma calcium and downregulates PTH secretion inappropriately. Inactivating mutations cause an increase in plasma calcium with elevated PTH levels because the calcium receptor is relatively insensitive.

It is not clear whether phosphate also has a role in regulating PTH secretion, with high concentrations stimulating secretion. This effect may also be an indirect consequence of the high phosphate levels causing a reduction in serum calcium concentration. PTH secretion is inhibited by calcitriol (see below).

As a peptide, PTH has a very short half-life in blood of around 5 minutes and is mostly metabolized in the liver and kidney, with the peptide fragments being excreted in the urine.

Actions of parathyroid hormone

Parathyroid hormone has two target tissues: kidney and bone. The main target tissue of PTH is the kidney where

PTH has three effects: first, to increase the reabsorption of calcium from urine; second, to increase the expression of the enzyme 1α-hydroxylase, which activates vitamin D (Fig. 12.6); and third, to increase the excretion of phosphate.

PTH, as a peptide, acts on cell surface G-protein coupled receptors. There are two forms of the PTH receptor, one of which also binds a related peptide called PTHrp (parathyroid hormone related peptide) and is termed the PTH-1 receptor. The other binds exclusively PTH and is the PTH-2 receptor. The receptors belong to a subfamily of G-protein coupled receptors which includes the ACTH receptor and act by stimulating both cAMP production and phospholipase C activation (see Ch. 2). Measurement of cAMP in urine can be used as an indication of PTH activity. PTH is a fast-acting hormone, causing a decrease in urinary calcium levels within a few minutes.

The second major target tissue for PTH is bone (see above) where PTH has different effects depending on both the concentration of PTH and duration of exposure to the cells. Low levels of PTH stimulate osteoblasts and bone formation whereas prolonged high levels of PTH increase osteoclast activity, causing an increase in bone resorption.

Parathyroid hormone related peptide (PTHrp)

PTHrp is structurally closely related to PTH and both peptides have equal affinity for the PTH-1 receptor.

Case 12.1 Primary hyperparathyroidism: 3

Case note: Test results

The investigations revealed:

Creatinine	112 mmol/L (normal <120 mmol/L)
Serum phosphate	0.8 mmol/L (normal 0.8–1.2 mmol/L)
Albumin	42 g/L (normal 36–48 g/L)
Serum calcium	3.45 mmol/L
Corrected serum calcium	3.41 mmol/L (normal 2.2–2.6 mmol/L)
Thyroid function, electrolytes, glucose	Normal
Alkaline phosphatase	220 U/L (normal <120 U/L)
Liver function tests	Normal
Abdominal radiography	Extensive faeces throughout colon and calcification over renal areas
Urine microbiology	Normal

What other test is needed to work out what has gone wrong with calcium homeostasis?

Mrs Smith has a high serum calcium level and the main acute regulator of serum calcium homeostasis is parathyroid hormone (PTH). PTH secretion from the parathyroid glands is normally stimulated by hypocalcaemia and inhibited by hypercalcaemia. So the further investigation was to measure serum PTH, which was abnormal at 15 pmol/L (normal range 1.2–6.7 pmol/L). Because PTH should normally be inhibited by the high serum calcium concentration, this suggests that the parathyroid glands are autonomously producing excessive PTH, which has caused the hypercalcaemia. PTH causes hypercalcaemia by acting on the kidneys and bone to mobilize calcium. The high alkaline phosphatase level is a marker of bone turnover.

While PTH is secreted exclusively by the cells of the parathyroid gland, the gene encoding PTHrp is expressed in a wide range of tissues and is frequently co-expressed with the PTH-1 receptor gene, suggesting that this peptide usually acts as a paracrine or autocrine messenger, rather than as a hormone. The one known hormonal effect of PTHrp is in disease: PTHrp is well-recognized as being the mediator of hypercalcaemia of malignancy (see below) and is commonly secreted by tumours of the lung, breast and kidney.

The normal physiological actions of PTHrp are less clear, but it appears to have developmental effects on fetal bone, effects on vascular smooth muscle, differentiation of breast tissue and of hair follicles in skin, and a role in the inflammatory response. PTHrp also appears to have a role in regulating calcium transport across the placenta. These actions all appear to be local effects rather than hormonal.

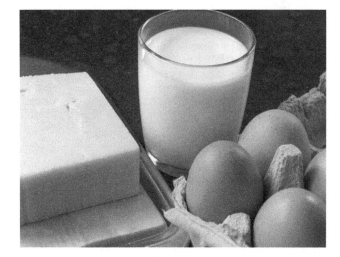

Figure 12.7 Dietary sources of vitamin D. Dairy products (shown) are good sources of vitamin D, as are fish and some meat, particularly liver. Vitamin D is added as a supplement to margarines.

Calcitriol: source and activation of vitamin D

There are two forms of vitamin D. The first is vitamin D3 (cholecalciferol), which can be made in the skin or derived from dietary sources such as dairy produce, oily fish and liver (Fig. 12.7). The second type of vitamin D is vitamin D2 (ergocalciferol), which is derived from yeast and fungi and is added to margarines as a food supplement. Both are activated to form calcitriol, and the two forms of calcitriol are equipotent. As there is little difference between vitamins D2 and D3, they are usually just referred to as 'vitamin D'. Similarly, because the two forms of calcitriol, one made from D2 and the other from D3, have identical effects, they are normally just referred to as 'calcitriol'.

Calcitriol has an important role in the long-term regulation of plasma calcium levels and is the activated form of vitamin D, a steroid derivative. Calcitriol is an unusual hormone in that it is not produced by a single gland or cell type and it is regulated in a different way from most hormones.

Vitamin D, the precursor of calcitriol, can either be obtained from the diet or made in the skin, by the action of sunlight (Fig. 12.8). The conversion of 7-dehydrocholesterol, known as pre-vitamin D, to vitamin D3 requires

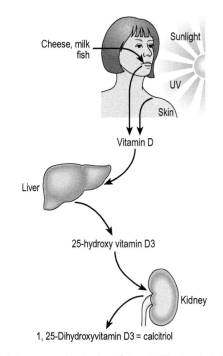

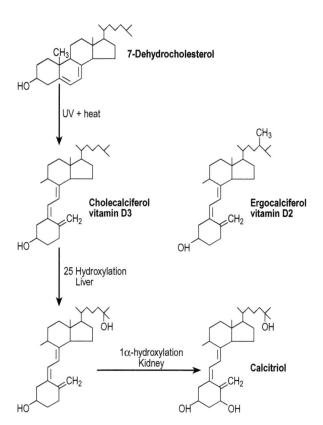

Figure 12.8 Sources and activation of vitamin D3. Vitamin D is obtained either from the skin through the action of sunlight, or from the diet. It is relatively inactive until it has been hydroxylated twice; the first reaction takes place in the liver and the second in the kidney, leading to the formation of the active hormone, calcitriol. UV, ultraviolet light.

Figure 12.9 Formation and structure of vitamin D3 (cholecalciferol) and D2 (ergocalciferol), and the formation of calcitriol. UV, ultraviolet light.

both light and heat. The optimal wavelength for production is 297 nm—in the ultraviolet range. Following the action of sunlight, the pre-vitamin D needs to remain in the warm skin for a while until the vitamin D is formed. The cells that produce vitamin D3 are in the lower layers of the skin, beneath the cells containing the pigment, melanin. This means that individuals with a high skin melanin content need a longer exposure to sunlight in order to produce the same amount of vitamin D3 as individuals with a lower melanin content. Overall, the amount of vitamin D3 entering the body depends principally on the amount of sun exposure and an individual's skin colour, although some is also absorbed from the diet. Vitamin D2 is absorbed from the gut and so the amount entering the body depends on an individual's diet.

It would be very unusual if the production of a hormone was not closely regulated, and clearly the supply of vitamin D to the body is not regulated. However, both vitamin D2 and D3 are relatively inactive and must undergo a process of chemical conversion to calcitriol in order to have significant effect (Fig. 12.9). It is this conversion process that is actively regulated. There are two steps in the activation of vitamin D, both hydroxylation reactions. The first step is a 25-hydroxylation, which occurs in the liver and is not regulated. The second step is 1α-hydroxylation, catalysed by a member of the *CYP* family of steroid hydroxylases, *CYP27B1*, which

is expressed in the kidney (Fig. 12.9). The expression of *CYP27B1* is actively regulated by PTH. The final active product of vitamin D activation is calcitriol.

Interesting fact

Do not be confused by the naming of this hormone, because it is known by several different names, although calcitriol is the easiest to remember. Vitamin D3 is properly known as cholecalciferol and so the active form, following the two hydroxylations, is 1,25-dihydroxycholecalciferol. It is also sometimes called 'active vitamin D3'. So 1,25-dihydroxycholecalciferol = 1,25-dihydroxyvitamin D = calcitriol. Likewise 1,25-dihydroxyergocalciferol = 1,25-dihydroxyvitamin D = calcitriol.

Vitamin D and calcitriol in blood

Vitamin D, formed in the skin or absorbed in the gut, binds to a vitamin D binding protein in blood. It has only a short half-life in blood as it is rapidly converted to 25-hydroxyvitamin D in the liver. This compound has a half-life of about 2 weeks and so provides a readily accessible reserve of hormone precursor in the blood. However, the active hormone, calcitriol, has a short half-life of just a few hours.

Interesting fact

Vitamin D3 is not really a vitamin. Vitamins are generally defined as organic compounds necessary for the correct functioning of the body but which the body cannot synthesize and so must be obtained from the diet. In most people adequate amounts of vitamin D3 can be synthesized in the body. Vitamin D3 is not a hormone either. It is not active until it has been metabolized to form calcitriol. Vitamin D3 should probably be classified as a hormone precursor.

Actions of calcitriol

As a steroid derivative, calcitriol acts on intracellular receptors to alter the rate of transcription of certain genes. Calcitriol receptors are called vitamin D receptors, VDR, and are members of the second class of nuclear receptors, related to thyroid hormone receptors but distinct from other steroid receptors. After binding calcitriol the VDR is phosphorylated, which enables it to recruit its preferred dimerization partner, the retinoic acid receptor (RXR), before binding to vitamin D response elements (VDREs) in the promoter region of the target gene (Fig. 12.10). There are often multiple VDREs in promoter regions and the VDR is able to inhibit transcription of certain genes and promote transcription of others. Vitamin D receptors are expressed in many tissues of the body including skin, bone, immune system, muscle (both skeletal and cardiac), and endocrine tissues. The effects of calcitriol are generally long-term regulatory actions, mediated by transcriptional changes in the target cell.

Effects on plasma calcium and bone

Calcitriol acts on cells in the gastrointestinal tract to increase the production of calcium transport proteins, termed calbindin-D proteins, which results in increased uptake of calcium from the gut into the body. This is the only mechanism by which the body can increase its calcium stores.

The actions of calcitriol on bone are not well understood but it is essential for normal osteoblast differentiation and function. It has a minor effect on the kidney, decreasing urinary loss of calcium by stimulating reabsorption. Calcitriol acts directly on the parathyroid gland, regulating calcium receptor levels and directly inhibiting transcription of the gene encoding PTH. Calcitriol also has important secondary effects on PTH secretion. By increasing calcium uptake in the gastrointestinal system, calcitriol increases plasma calcium, maintaining PTH secretion at low levels and thus favouring osteoblast action and protecting bone structure.

Effects on the immune system

It is clear that vitamin D is necessary for a healthy immune system. It has been known for many years that individuals with vitamin D deficiency are more prone to

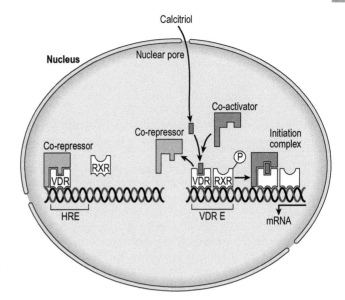

Figure 12.10 Molecular action of calcitriol. Calcitriol binds to vitamin D receptors (VDR) which are located in the nucleus of target cells. Binding of the calcitriol causes the VDR to become phosphorylated which allows it to recruit the retinoic acid receptor (RXR) to form a dimer which binds to the vitamin D response element (VDRE) in a gene promoter. The dimer attracts co-activators to form an initiation complex and permit gene transcription to proceed.

infection. There is good evidence that chronic vitamin D deficiency is associated with increased incidence of autoimmune diseases.

The VDR is expressed in all the cell types in the immune system, including T lymphocytes and macrophages. There is a two-way communication between vitamin D and the immune system: immune mediators act on the kidney to increase expression of the *CYP27B1* gene, which encodes the 1α-hydroxylase enzyme responsible for activation of vitamin D3.

Calcitriol has a wide range of actions in the immune system. It acts directly on T cells and modulates their function. It also enhances the antimicrobial activity of macrophages and monocytes by increasing release of antimicrobial agents.

Effects on cancer

Several studies have shown that there is an inverse relationship between sunlight exposure and cancer mortality. Epidemiological studies have also found that a higher intake of vitamin D3 or greater exposure to sunlight is associated with lower overall risk of developing cancer. It is known that calcitriol has several effects which together function to inhibit cancer growth. Calcitriol causes an increase in the length of the cell cycle so that the rate of cell division of cancerous cells is slowed. It increases the rate of apoptosis, programmed cell death, and inhibits angiogenesis, the formation of new blood vessels, which is important for tumour survival. Furthermore, calcitriol inhibits the breakdown of the extracellular matrix around tumours and so inhibits the formation of metastases. It seems that vitamin D may be a useful agent in the treatment of some forms of cancer, but whether vitamin D supplementation is a useful preventive measure is still not clear.

Therapeutic uses of vitamin D3

Until recently, the only therapeutic use of vitamin D3 was as a replacement therapy in individuals with low endogenous vitamin D3 levels and in postmenopausal women to prevent osteoporosis. The recent studies suggesting beneficial effects in some forms of cancer have resulted in a proliferation of websites offering vitamin D3 for sale, claiming that it will cure cancer, inflammatory diseases and all the world's ills. One issue is that long-term use of high levels of vitamin D is associated with hypercalcaemia, so a lot of effort is going into the development of analogues that will exert immunomodulatory effects and anti-cancer effects without the associated effects on calcium metabolism. There is evidence that vitamin D may be an effective immunosuppressant for long-term use in autoimmune disorders and following organ transplantation. Recently, vitamin D has become a first-line treatment for the hyperproliferative skin condition, psoriasis, often used in combination with a glucocorticoid. It has been suggested that vitamin D may be cardioprotective and exert an anti-aging effect on both muscle and brain, but there is not yet enough evidence to support its use as an anti-aging therapy. However, it is clear that the biology and therapeutic uses of vitamin D are an important and fast-moving area of endocrinology.

Effects of other hormones on plasma calcium

Glucocorticoids, growth hormone, thyroid hormones and insulin all affect plasma calcium and bone physiology to some extent. Insulin-like growth factor-I is produced in bone in response to growth hormone stimulation, and acts to stimulate bone formation, as does insulin itself. Growth hormone causes an increase in renal calcium excretion, but also appears to stimulate gastrointestinal absorption of calcium. Glucocorticoids inhibit osteoclast activity in the short term and so decrease plasma calcium but over a longer period of time they cause a decrease in bone formation and an increase in resorption, resulting in osteoporosis. Glucocorticoids also decrease calcium uptake in the gut and increase renal excretion of both calcium and phosphate.

Excess secretion of thyroid hormones can cause bone loss resulting in hypercalcaemia and increased urinary excretion of calcium.

Disorders of hypercalcaemia

The physiological response to hypercalcaemia is shown in Figure 12.11. In general, any excess calcium in blood is simply excreted in the urine and hypercalcaemia is relatively uncommon. There are two major pathological causes of high serum calcium levels. Oversecretion of PTH, as in the clinical case, may result from a parathyroid adenoma and is termed primary hyperparathyroidism. The second major cause of hypercalcaemia is cancer related. Various cancers produce a peptide, called parathyroid hormone-related peptide (PTHrp), which has very similar actions to PTH and causes 'hypercalcaemia of malignancy' and suppression of PTH secretion. There may also be hypercalcaemia as a result of metastases in bone causing an increased rate of bone breakdown. Rarely, very high levels of calcium-carrying proteins in the circulation may result in a falsely increased total serum calcium level, when the free or ionized calcium concentration is normal.

Case 12.1 **Primary hyperparathyroidism: 4**

Case note: Explanation
An understanding of calcium physiology helps in understanding the symptoms. Urinary symptoms tend to occur early in the evolution of the disease. Serum calcium is filtered in the urine and, at high levels, acts as an osmotic diuretic. Thus, in Mrs Smith, the high level of calcium in the urine increased the volume of the urine and led to nocturia. Calcium also came out of solution and formed stones. This resulted in renal colic. Hypertension was a consequence of the long exposure of the kidneys to high calcium levels.

When serum calcium levels are higher, abdominal and general symptoms occur. Calcium is important for nerve and muscle function. The muscle of the gut fails to contract properly when the calcium level is too high, resulting in constipation. Depression and tiredness are cerebral effects of high calcium levels.

Very high serum calcium levels (as in parathyroid storm) may lead to cardiorespiratory failure, coma and death. This is a serious risk if the patient is dehydrated. More commonly, as in this case, adenoma of one or more of the parathyroid glands results in an insidious increase in calcium levels and symptoms over many years.

Following investigation to locate the abnormal parathyroid gland, Mrs Smith underwent successful surgery (parathyroidectomy) and made a complete recovery.

Interesting fact

A useful way of remembering the symptoms of hypercalcaemia:

- Stones (kidney stones)
- Moans (depression)
- Groans (abdominal pains).

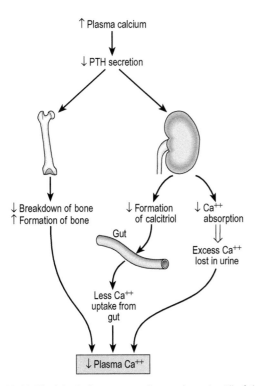

Figure 12.11 Physiological response to hypercalcaemia. All of the mechanisms designed to conserve calcium are switched off, and the excess calcium is excreted in the urine.

Treatment

The treatment of primary hyperparathyroidism is initially to give fluids to restore the circulating volume and make up for losses of urine. Definitive treatment is parathyroidectomy to remove a usually benign tumour of one of the four parathyroid glands. The affected gland is identified using either ultrasonography or sestamibi imaging (Fig. 12.12).

Effects of excess vitamin D

Excess circulating vitamin D does not occur from the actions of sunlight on skin, it is always a consequence of ingestion of excess vitamin D. The acute effects are nausea, headaches, weakness and lethargy. There is a significant rise in circulating calcium which is excreted in the urine resulting in osmotic diuresis and polyuria. Chronic vitamin D excess causes the formation of kidney stones and may cause calcification of blood vessels. It is treated by removing the source of vitamin D and by treating with glucocorticoids, which antagonize the effects of calcitriol on gastrointestinal calcium uptake. It can take several weeks for the body to eliminate the excess vitamin D.

Disorders of hypocalcaemia

The physiological response to hypocalcaemia is shown in Figure 12.13. This regulatory system is totally dependent on an adequate supply of dietary calcium. If there is

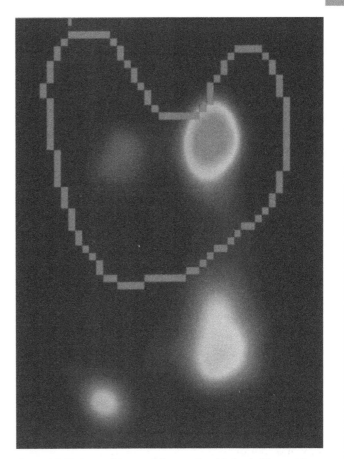

Figure 12.12 Sestamibi scan of the parathyroid glands. The position of all four parathyroid glands is shown by scanning after uptake of radiolabelled sestamibi. Note that the left upper parathyroid gland is particularly enlarged in this patient suffering from multiple endocrine neoplasia. The outline of the thyroid gland is shown.

a chronic lack of adequate calcium uptake from the diet, then the body sacrifices bone in order to maintain plasma calcium concentrations within the normal range. For this reason it is usually possible to maintain serum calcium within the normal concentration range, however severe the dietary calcium deficiency may be.

Vitamin D deficiency

The most common reason for lack of effective calcium uptake in the gut is vitamin D deficiency. This results from a combination of a diet lacking meat, fish and dairy products, and a lack of adequate exposure to sunlight. It may also be seen in chronic renal failure, as the damaged kidney is no longer able to effectively perform 1-hydroxylation to produce 1,25-hydroxyvitamin D (calcitriol).

The bone-sacrificing effect is seen in cases of vitamin D deficiency in adults, which results in osteomalacia (see below). In children this is seen as rickets. In vitamin D deficiency, the compensation by increased secretion of PTH can make it possible for the body to maintain serum calcium levels within the normal range, and in chronic cases this can lead to a secondary hyperparathyroidism.

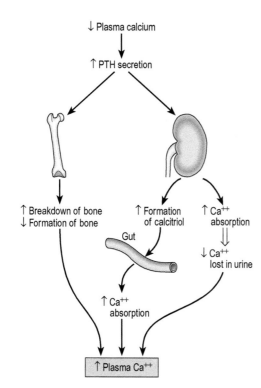

Figure 12.13 Physiological response to hypocalcaemia. The emphasis is on maintaining plasma calcium concentrations even if this results in loss of bone mass. The only way to increase total body calcium levels is through increased uptake of dietary calcium.

Interesting fact

In the UK, during the Second World War, chalk (calcium carbonate) was added to all flour and vitamin D was added to margarine in order to prevent rickets, which had been prevalent up to that time. Rickets had previously been treated (although not prevented) with cod liver oil—not very popular among the children required to take it. The staple diet of many poor, malnourished inner city communities was bread and margarine, so these were the most obvious foods to supplement. Since that time many food laws have been passed, but all still require the supplementation of all flour with calcium carbonate, and of margarine with vitamin D. In the USA, vitamin D is added to milk.

Parathyroid hormone deficiency

In the case of PTH deficiency, normal plasma calcium levels cannot be achieved. Hypoparathyroidism is uncommon, but causes serious and life-threatening hypocalcaemia. Without PTH it is not possible to maintain normal plasma calcium levels. Surgical removal of all the parathyroid glands causes symptoms of hypocalcaemia to appear within 48h. The consequences of hypocalcaemia include hyperexcitability of the neuromuscular junction, which causes paraesthesiae (pins and needles), tetanic contractions of skeletal muscle and even convulsions. When the respiratory muscles are affected this causes death. This hypocalcaemic *tetany* is not to be confused with *tetanus* caused by toxins produced by the bacterium *Clostridium tetani*.

Diseases of bone

Osteoporosis

Osteoporosis is a disease characterized by low bone mass and micro-architectural deterioration of bone tissue. This leads to bone fragility and a greatly increased fracture risk. In particular, there is a tendency for the bone to fracture in response to a relatively minor trauma. It is a disorder that affects one in five men but one in two women. It is therefore a significant public health problem. There are two reasons why women are more susceptible to osteoporosis than men: first, women have a lower peak bone mass than men; and second, they have an accelerated rate of bone loss after the menopause. Hormone replacement therapy (HRT) used to be considered a preventive treatment for osteoporosis, but the side-effects of long-term HRT use mean that it is now considered unsuitable. Lifestyle is considered to be an important factor in preventing osteoporosis, with a diet rich in vitamin D and calcium recommended together with exercise to help maintain healthy bones. In cases where osteoporosis is diagnosed, bisphosphonates are used to treat the disorder. These drugs act by suppressing osteoclast activity. They do this in two ways: by directly inhibiting recruitment of new osteoclasts and by stimulating osteoblasts to produce an osteoclast inhibitor.

Osteomalacia and rickets

Osteomalacia occurs when there is insufficient calcium (or phosphate) to mineralize newly formed bone. So a loss of bone mineral density is seen, with a greatly increased risk of fracture. In children, who are still in the phase of bone growth, vitamin D deficiency results in insufficient calcium being available both to maintain serum levels and for normal bone growth. This results in a failure of bone mineralization, leading to deformation of bones, particularly the long bones, in a condition called rickets. Although rickets is now uncommon, it used to be a major feature of large industrial cities where poor diet, combined with lack of exposure to sunlight, resulted in many children having vitamin D deficiency.

Paget's disease

Paget's disease, like osteoporosis, is a disease of older age that results in marked increases in bone fractures. Paget's disease is a poorly understood condition characterized by a marked increase in turnover in certain bones within the skeleton, while other bones remain unaffected.

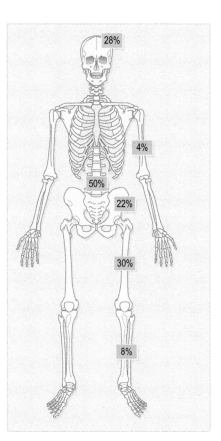

Figure 12.14 Diagram showing the parts of the skeleton most likely to be affected by Paget's disease (from Chew S L, Leslie D. 2006. Clinical endocrinology and diabetes: an illustrated colour text. Churchill Livingstone, Edinburgh, with permission).

Paget's disease may affect only one bone or several (Fig. 12.14). It is a disease of osteoclasts, which are abnormally large and cause an increase in bone resorption. This triggers osteoblasts, which are normal, to form new bone. However, the new bone is structurally disorganized, resulting in pain and increased fracture risk. It is thought to affect about 2% of the population aged over 55 years, but often occurs without symptoms. Treatment is usually with bisphosphonates.

A brief mention of calcitonin

Calcitonin is usually included in endocrine textbooks as the third hormone involved in the regulation of plasma calcium. It is a peptide hormone of 32 amino acids, secreted by the parafollicular cells of the thyroid gland and is considered to be a calcium-lowering hormone. Its physiological role is doubtful, however, because of the total lack of pathology resulting from either hyper- or hypo-secretion of calcitonin. It has been suggested that this peptide may have a role in pregnancy and lactation to preserve the maternal skeleton, but otherwise its actions appear to be confined to lower vertebrates.

Interesting fact

Although calcitonin does not appear to be physiologically important in humans, it does have a therapeutic use. Subcutaneous injection of salmon calcitonin was the first widely used treatment for Paget's disease. It was found to halve bone turnover and improve symptoms. Its use today is limited mostly to patients who cannot tolerate bisphosphonates.

Regulation of serum phosphate

Phosphate is not as tightly regulated as serum calcium. However, there is a degree of co-regulation of calcium and phosphate. Vitamin D stimulates the uptake of both calcium and phosphate in the gut and kidney. The actions of both vitamin D and PTH on bone also cause an increase in serum phosphate levels. However, there is clear divergent regulation of calcium and phosphate in the kidney in response to PTH, which stimulates reabsorption of calcium but excretion of phosphate. This is because the likelihood of calcium phosphate crystals forming is dependent on the product of calcium concentration and phosphate concentration. If phosphate concentrations increase then calcium phosphate stones are more likely to occur in the kidney. Therefore the actions of PTH tend to keep this product fairly constant.

MISCELLANEOUS HORMONES

13

Chapter objectives

After studying this chapter you should be able to:

1. Understand the role of erythropoietin in preventing anaemia.

2. Understand the role of the pineal gland and melatonin.

3. Appreciate the interactions between paracrine factors and hormones that control blood pressure.

4. Appreciate the complexity of interaction between the immune and endocrine systems, including the nature and roles of cytokines.

5. Appreciate the hormonal changes that occur with ageing.

6. Describe the principal endocrine components in the regulation of appetite.

The previous chapters of this book have dealt with the major endocrine systems of the body and their associated disorders. There are several other hormones that have not been covered and some processes that are controlled by an interaction between different systems. This chapter aims to cover the odds and ends of endocrinology and to consider some integrated systems, such as the regulation of blood pressure and volume, and the hormonal regulation of appetite.

Case 13.1 Progressive anaemia: 1

Case history

Mr Singh, a 55-year-old man with a long history of progressive chronic renal failure, is seen in outpatients for routine review. The cause of his kidney disease is chronic glomerulonephritis and the disease process can only be slowed down by good control of blood pressure. His serum creatinine level has risen from 210 mmol/L 2 years ago (estimated glomerular filtration rate (GFR) 33 mL/min) to 268 mmol/L 1 year ago (estimated GFR 28 mL/min) to 303 mmol/L at present (estimated GFR 24 mL/min).

His haemoglobin (Hb) level has fallen during recent months:

12 months ago	Hb 12.0 g/dL
6 months ago	Hb 13.4 g/dL
Today	Hb 10.6 g/dL

Other results:

Ferritin	243 ng/mL (normal)
B12 and folate	Normal
White cell and platelet counts	Normal

What is the most likely cause of Mr Singh's anaemia? How would you treat it?

Erythropoietin

We shall start by looking at a hormone produced by the kidney. We have already seen that the kidney is a target tissue for arginine vasopressin (AVP), aldosterone and parathyroid hormone (PTH), and that it controls the activation of vitamin D. However, the kidney is also an endocrine gland, producing a peptide hormone called erythropoietin (EPO or epo, pronounced 'E.P.O.' and 'eepo', respectively).

Erythropoietin is a glycosylated peptide hormone secreted by the fibroblasts adjacent to the renal tubules. It is secreted in response to either hypoxia or anaemia, but secretion is impaired in renal failure.

Erythropoietin is classified as a cytokine (see below) and acts through a specific receptor which is a member of the cytokine receptor family, linked to protein phosphorylation through JAK-STAT activation (see Ch. 2).

The major action of erythropoietin is on the bone marrow, where it stimulates the formation of red blood cells by preventing apoptosis of erythrocyte precursor cells. An erythropoietin deficiency results in fewer red cells that contain normal amounts of iron and are a normal shape and size—in other words, a normochromic, normocytic anaemia.

Increasingly, treatment for renal failure includes replacement therapy with recombinant erythropoietin. This is indicated when other causes of anaemia, such as iron, B12 or folate deficiency, have been ruled out.

Interesting fact

It has been recognized for many years that athletes can boost their red blood cell count by training at high altitudes, where the oxygen pressure is lower, causing erythropoietin stimulation. With a higher concentration of red blood cells, athletes participating in endurance sports, such as long-distance running or cycling, will be at an advantage. More recently, with the development of recombinant erythropoietin, some athletes bypassed the altitude training and simply injected erythropoietin to boost their red blood cells. In several cases this led to pathological levels of red blood cell production (polycythaemia), resulting in stroke and thrombosis. This is likely to explain the sudden deaths of a number of athletes over recent years.

Case 13.1 Progressive anaemia: 2

Case note: Treatment

Mr Singh's anaemia is likely to be caused by erythropoietin deficiency as a direct consequence of his renal failure. The test results indicate that it is not due to iron, B12 or folate deficiency.

He will be started on treatment with one of the forms of erythropoietin currently available. Treatment begins with a low dose and is varied over several weeks until the target Hb concentration of around 11–13 g/dL is reached. Erythropoietin is a peptide hormone, so must be given by injection. The different forms of erythropoietin have different durations of action, but treatment is typically given one to three times per week. It is also important to ensure that Mr Singh has adequate iron stores or the erythropoietin will not be as effective.

Immune–endocrine interactions: cytokines and eicosanoids

Previous chapters in this book have briefly mentioned some interactions between the immune and endocrine systems, including the effects of glucocorticoids on inflammatory and immune processes and the effects of autoimmune disease on the thyroid and pancreas. These are examples of the more obvious manifestations of the significant and complex interactions between the immune and endocrine systems. In order to look more closely at this we need to consider some of the molecules involved.

Cytokines

Cells of the immune system produce a range of chemical messengers called cytokines. However, it is not just immune cells that secrete cytokines: they are also made in vascular endothelial cells, the liver, adipocytes and many other tissues. The cytokines are families of peptides that include interleukins, erythropoietin, interferons, bone morphogenetic proteins (BMPs) and several families of growth factors, including insulin-like growth factor-1 (IGF-1) which mediates many of the effects of growth hormone, as we saw in Chapter 4. More than 100 cytokines have been identified to date.

These cytokines can act in an endocrine, paracrine or autocrine manner to bring about their effects, mediated by specific receptors, mostly of the single-transmembrane domain class, which act by activation of the Janus kinase (JAK)-STAT pathway (see Ch. 2). The different cytokines have a wide range of effects on the immune system, stimulating activation of lymphocytes and macrophages and promoting differentiation of B cells and eosinophils. Although cytokines were originally identified as messengers within the immune system, they have a somewhat broader range of effects than this, particularly in fetal development and cellular differentiation.

Cytokines also have a role in the regulation of endocrine systems. They have been implicated in the acute regulation of hormone secretion, including the release of hypothalamic stimulating factors, particularly in the response to exercise and stress. Cytokines are also known to regulate the expression of steroid-metabolizing enzymes and to have a major role in ovarian follicle maturation. They also have a longer-term role in the growth and differentiation of every endocrine tissue. It is becoming increasingly clear that cytokines are ubiquitous signalling molecules and have effects on every tissue in the body, including the endocrine system. The possibility of exploiting cytokines therapeutically is very exciting, and they are already used in the treatment of some cancers. We do not yet know how the actions of cytokines may be used in the management of endocrine disorders, and much research will be required to advance this field, but there is clearly a great deal of potential in the clinical application of cytokine research.

Eicosanoids

Some cytokines, such as interleukin-1, have a role in the promotion of inflammation. In this role, they interact with a family of signalling molecules termed eicosanoids. The eicosanoids include prostaglandins, prostacyclins, thromboxanes and leukotrienes, which are all synthesized from membrane phospholipids via arachidonic acid (Fig. 13.1). Prostaglandins were given this name because they were first isolated from semen and found to be secreted by the prostate gland. It is now known that eicosanoid synthesis takes place in virtually all tissues of the body. It is known that the eicosanoids produced by the actions of one of the cyclo-oxygenase enzymes, COX2, are those most involved in pain and inflammation, so a range of drugs has been developed to specifically inhibit COX2.

In addition to their well recognized role as inflammatory mediators, the eicosanoids have several other functions, including a role in endocrine regulation, principally in the female reproductive system. In the ovary, there is a rise in prostaglandin synthesis in the pre-ovulatory follicle, with the pre-ovulatory burst of luteinizing hormone increasing COX2 expression and so stimulating the release of prostaglandins E2 and F2a from follicular granulosa cells. This increase in COX2 expression and prostaglandin synthesis is now known to be an essential step in ovulation, and it has been shown that rupture of the follicle and release of the oocyte can be prevented by non-steroidal anti-inflammatory drugs (NSAIDs), which inhibit cyclo-oxygenase enzymes (Fig. 13.1). In the light of this knowledge, women who are attempting to become pregnant are advised to avoid taking both non-selective NSAIDs and the selective COX2 inhibitors. Prostaglandins are also thought to have a role in fertilization and implantation of the embryo. In addition, prostaglandins are important in parturition as they cause ripening and dilatation of the cervix. When labour is induced, prostaglandin pessaries are used as part of the treatment.

In seminal fluid, the high concentrations of prostaglandins are thought to have an immunosuppressive effect on the female reproductive tract, allowing the sperm to reach the uterus without triggering an immune response. It has been suggested that blocking prostaglandin

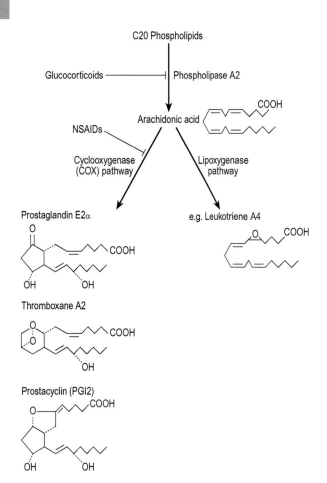

Figure 13.1 The eicosanoids are synthesized from phospholipids in the cell membrane via the production of arachidonic acid. The action of phospholipase A2 on lipids such as linoleic acid releases arachidonic acid. The arachidonic acid is metabolized by groups of enzymes called cyclo-oxygenases or lipoxygenases to release prostaglandins, thromboxanes and leukotrienes. The structures of some of these compounds are shown.

production by use of NSAIDs has an adverse effect on sperm quality. It has also been suggested that the age-related decline in testosterone production by Leydig cells may be related to the increased expression of COX enzymes in the testes with increasing age.

Prostacyclin and thromboxane both have a significant role in the local regulation of vascular tone, with prostacyclin acting as a vasodilator whereas thromboxane vasoconstricts (see below). They also have opposing actions on platelet aggregation, with thromboxane promoting platelet aggregation and clot formation, while prostacyclin inhibits this process.

Age-related changes in hormone secretion

It is well known that women go through the menopause at around the age of 50 years and may experience adverse effects of the associated decrease in oestrogen secretion, but the age-related decrease in other hormones is much less recognized. Men do not go through any process comparable to the menopause, but there is an age-related decline in testosterone secretion, and some men experience hypogonadal symptoms associated with this. Perhaps predictably this has been termed *andropause*. The growth hormone (GH)–IGF axis also shows a marked decrease with age, a phenomenon termed *somatopause*, and, to complete the set, the adrenocortical secretion of its major androgen, dehydroepiandrosterone (DHEA), also declines with age—termed *adrenopause*.

It is not clear why age-related changes to these specific endocrine systems occur. There are no comparable patterns of change in thyroid function, for example, and the adrenopause does not include significant decreases in cortisol or aldosterone secretion.

It has been suggested that the mechanisms of andropause and somatopause might be linked, with an intact GH–IGF axis required for appropriate testicular function and an appropriate level of testosterone required to support GH secretion, but there is little evidence to support this suggestion.

Hormone replacement therapy in ageing

There are plenty of websites offering to sell you anti-ageing hormone treatments. DHEA, testosterone and GH are all readily available. But is there any evidence that they will keep you fit and healthy in old age? For most treatments the answer is 'no'. Unless somebody has a properly diagnosed hormone deficiency then there is no benefit at all in taking 'replacement therapy'. Hormone replacement therapy for postmenopausal women is well established, and testosterone replacement therapy for men with hypogonadism of old age is also a routine part of clinical practice. Administration of GH to older people who do not have a defined GH deficiency is associated with a number of adverse effects, including carpal tunnel syndrome. Probably the most popular and potentially least harmful hormonal anti-ageing treatment is DHEA. In the USA, DHEA is available over the counter and appears to be taken by a large number of individuals in a huge uncontrolled and unsupervised experiment. Although there appear to be very few side-effects from taking DHEA, other than greasy skin and acne, it does not appear to have any major beneficial effects either.

Melatonin

Melatonin is a hormone involved in regulating circadian rhythms. It is produced by the pineal gland—a small gland in the brain, named because it is the size and shape of a pine nut. Melatonin was discovered by Lerner in 1958 when he was looking for the hormone that controls

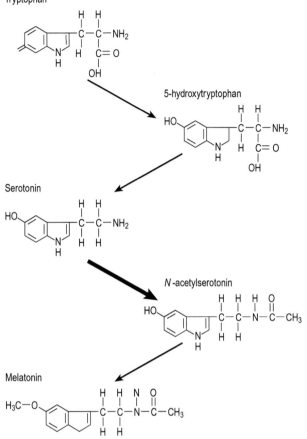

Figure 13.2 Synthesis of melatonin. The rate-limiting step is the conversion of serotonin to *N*-acetylserotonin, shown by the heavy arrow.

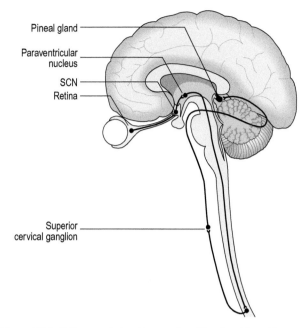

Figure 13.3 Pathways of pineal innervation. The signal from the retina is relayed through the suprachiasmatic nucleus (SCN) and the paraventricular nucleus, down the spinal column, returning via the superior cervical ganglion to supply the pineal gland (from Wehr T A et al. 2001. Arch Gen Psychiatry 58:1108–1114, with permission of the American Medical Association).

melanin production in lizards. Melatonin is synthesized from tryptophan (Fig. 13.2) and its production is negatively controlled by light, so that light falling on the retina inhibits melatonin secretion. There is not a direct neural pathway from the retina to the pineal gland, but a rather complex reflex involving the cervical ganglion (Fig. 13.3). As a consequence, damage to the spinal column in this area can severely disrupt diurnal rhythms.

In humans there is a circadian rhythm of melatonin secretion, with levels being very low during the daylight hours and increasing from dusk until a peak is reached at around 0300 hours. Subsequently melatonin levels decline until daytime. This secretory pattern is controlled by a number of *zeitgebers* (time-givers), which include light, posture, social cues and melatonin itself. There is also a marked age dependency of melatonin secretion, with maximal secretion seen in early childhood, at around 3 years, and a gradual diminution of the amplitude of the nocturnal increase in melatonin secretion with advancing years.

The major role of melatonin is in regulating circadian rhythms of the body, including body temperature and the secretion of other hormones. It has been described as the 'circadian glue', responsible for holding the other biological rhythms in phase. In other animals, melatonin has a key role in regulating seasonal fertility by controlling the hypothalamo–pituitary–gonadal axis. There is some evidence that melatonin can affect luteinizing hormone and follicle stimulating hormone production in the human, and it has even been suggested that it may play a role in the timing of menarche, but the extent of its role remains unclear. There has been a lot of recent interest in both the antioxidant properties of melatonin and its complex interactions with the immune system. Although these functions are poorly understood, melatonin's potential as an immune modulator and in cancer treatment is being researched extensively.

Clinically, melatonin has been used in the treatment of sleep disorders in older people and in regulating the body clock of 'blind free-runners', a group of profoundly blind people whose body clock does not naturally follow the usual 24-hour cycle.

Interesting fact

In the USA melatonin, like DHEA, is classified as a foodstuff and so is freely available and marketed for its supposed health benefits, one of which is the treatment of jetlag. Given at an appropriate time, melatonin may be used to phase-advance or phase-delay the circadian clock (Fig. 13.4), as desired. However, both the dose and the timing of melatonin are critical for it to have an effect.

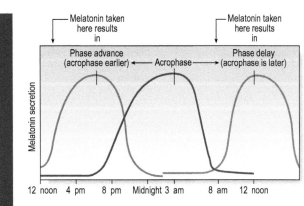

Figure 13.4 Use of melatonin to phase shift diurnal rhythms. Melatonin secretion is stimulated by nightfall, and reaches a maximum at about 0300 hours. When travelling through time zones, melatonin administration can be used to phase-advance or phase-delay this secretion pattern, so resetting the biological clock for a different time zone.

Gut hormones

The first hormone to be discovered, in 1905, was a gut hormone, secretin. Over the past 100 years the study of endocrinology has flourished as we have characterized more hormones, and recognized their effects. That secretin was the first hormone to be discovered is somewhat paradoxical, as it is among the least important of all the hormones recognized today. Indeed, secretin is frequently relegated to a historical footnote in endocrine texts. Although secretin is recognized as an important gut hormone, regulating bicarbonate secretion from the pancreas, there is little pathology associated with this peptide, so it does not excite much interest. We now know that secretin is just one of a large number of polypeptide hormones secreted by cells of the gastrointestinal tract. These hormones, their major sites of production and their main physiological actions are summarized in Table 13.1. These hormones,

Table 13.1 Gastrointestinal hormones

Name	*Structure (No. of amino acids)*	*Main sites of production*	*Major actions*
Secretin family			
Secretin	27	S cells in duodenum and jejunum	↑ Bicarbonate secretion from pancreas
Glucagon	29	A cells in upper GI tract	↑ Plasma glucose
VIP	28	Nerves throughout GI tract	↑ Intestinal secretion of electrolytes and water into lumen of gut, relaxation of sphincters
Gastrin family			
CCK	39 (variously sized fragments)	I cells in duodenum	↑ Pancreatic enzyme secretion ↑ Contraction of gall bladder
Gastrin	34	G cells in antral portion of gastric mucosa	↑ Gastric acid and pepsin secretion
GIP	43	K cells in duodenum and jejunum	↑ Insulin secretion
Other hormones			
GRP	27	Vagal nerve endings on G cells	↑ Gastrin secretion
Motilin	22	Enterochromaffin cells and motilin-immunopositive cells in stomach, small intestine and colon	↑ Contraction of smooth muscle and promotes GI motility
Substance P	11	Neurons throughout GI tract	↑ Motility of small intestine
Guanylin	15	Cells of intestinal mucosa	↑ Cl⁻ secretion into gut lumen
Ghrelin	28	Stomach	Stimulates appetite
Neurotensin	13	Neurons in ileum	Inhibits GI motility ↑ Ileal blood flow
Somatostatin	14	D cells in gastrointestinal mucosa	↓ Secretion of gastrin, VIP and GIP

CCK, cholecystokinin; GI, gastrointestinal; GIP, gastric inhibitory peptide; GRP, gastrin releasing peptide; VIP, vasoactive intestinal polypeptide.

and the cells that produce them, are considered to be part of the 'diffuse endocrine system'. This term describes the myriad hormones secreted by endocrine and neuroendocrine cells that are scattered throughout the body, rather than being assembled into discrete endocrine glands.

Endocrine disorders involving these gastrointestinal hormones are relatively uncommon. Occasionally tumours of the gastrointestinal cells secreting these hormones are detected, but they are rare. The tumour most frequently seen is gastrin secreting, termed a gastrinoma, and causes Zollinger–Ellison syndrome. When a gastrinoma is detected, the patient is investigated for multiple endocrine neoplasia (MEN), a condition that is commonly found in patients presenting with gastrinoma (see below).

Other tumours include glucagonoma, somatostatinoma and VIPoma. The latter is interesting because it presents with high volumes of watery diarrhoea, sometimes exceeding 5 L/day. Surgical removal of the tumour is the usual treatment, although the synthetic somatostatin analogue, octreotide, may be used to treat excess vasoactive intestinal peptide (VIP) or gastrin secretion.

The hormonal control of appetite: fat is an endocrine tissue

Recently, with the increase in the incidence of obesity and the metabolic syndrome in the general population, there has been a huge interest in the possibility of using hormones to manipulate appetite pharmacologically. It was hoped that an appetite-suppressant drug could be developed that would make dieting easier. As a result of all the research effort, we now have an improved understanding of the hormonal signals that make us hungry and also tell us when we have eaten enough. The hormonal signals regulating appetite are summarized in Figure 13.5. There are hormones produced by the gut, the pancreas and by adipose tissue that tell the appetite centre in the brain that we do not need to eat. Perhaps the most interesting of these hormones is leptin, a peptide hormone produced by fat cells.

In previous chapters we have seen that adipose tissue (fat) has a role in the conversion of testosterone to oestradiol by the action of the enzyme aromatase, which is expressed in adipose tissue. Adipocytes also secrete peptide hormones, including a range of cytokines, and leptin, a peptide hormone involved in appetite regulation. The circulating concentration of leptin is directly proportional to the absolute mass of fat in the body. Synthesis of leptin is regulated by food intake and rises after a meal. On the other hand, leptin levels decrease with fasting and it is this decrease that signals hunger. One of the actions of leptin is to inhibit secretion of the hypothalamic hormones, orexins, which have a powerful stimulatory effect on appetite (Ch. 3). Several cases of people with a leptin deficiency have been described. These individuals have a raging hunger that is never satisfied, except by injection of leptin. In theory, it should be possible to

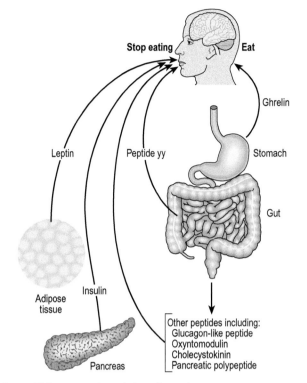

Figure 13.5 Hormonal regulation of appetite.

suppress appetite by administering leptin, but in practice this does not work. In obese individuals, there is already a high level of circulating leptin and injection of more leptin has little effect on appetite.

There have been recent clinical trials on peptide YY that have had promising results. People who had infusions of this peptide ate less than people infused with saline. The problem is that the peptide has to be injected, which is not very practical, and although it reduces the amount eaten at the next meal we do not know whether it will work over a longer period of time.

In endocrinology, having several hormones doing the same job tells you that the job is important, and we can certainly see that with appetite regulation. There is so much redundancy in this system that it is not surprising that we have not found a magic diet pill.

Interesting fact

There is growing evidence that there are endocrinological differences between adipose tissues in different parts of the body. In particular, adipocytes (fat cells) in subcutaneous fat (under the skin) appear to metabolize and synthesize steroid hormones differently from adipocytes in omental fat (in the abdominal cavity). It is already known that 'central obesity', with a high waist to hip ratio, is a better predictor of cardiovascular risk than total body fat. Research into the endocrinology of fat is an exciting and rapidly developing area.

Multiple organ disorders in endocrinology

Multiple endocrine neoplasia (MEN)

MEN is an inherited condition that affects approximately 1 in 10000 of the population. There are three distinct forms of MEN, with different characteristics (Table 13.2). MEN1 is also known as Wermer's syndrome and includes hyperparathyroidism in nearly all cases. In this condition there are often tumours of the gastrointestinal tract or pancreas, most commonly secreting gastrin or insulin. MEN2a, also known as Sipple's syndrome, nearly always features medullary carcinoma of the thyroid, with phaeochromocytoma seen in around half of the patients. MEN2b, also known as MEN3, is characterized by a high incidence of mucosal neuromas in addition to the medullary thyroid carcinoma characteristic of MEN2a.

Multiple endocrine neoplasia is difficult to treat. As well as the possibilities of multiple disorders simultaneously, the individual disorders are often complicated.

Table 13.2 Multiple endocrine neoplasia

Type	Features	(%)
MEN1	Parathyroid tumour	≈80
	Pancreatic tumour	≈75
	Pituitary tumour	≈65
MEN2a	Medullary thyroid carcinoma	≈100
	Phaeochromocytoma	≈50
	Parathyroid tumour	≈40
MEN2b (MEN3)	Mucosal neuroma	≈100
	Medullary thyroid carcinoma	≈100
	Phaeochromocytoma	≈45
	Parathyroid tumour	Rare

MEN1 is caused by a loss of function mutation of the MENIN tumour-suppressor gene on chromosome 11. MEN2a and 2b are both associated with activating mutations in the RET proto-oncogene on chromosome 10.

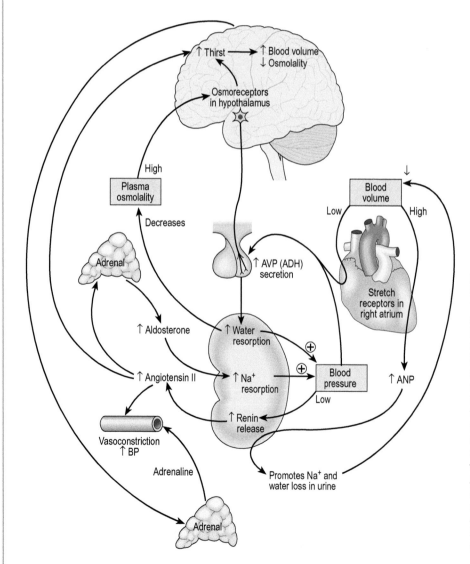

Figure 13.6 Hormonal regulation of blood pressure, volume and osmolality. There is a complex interaction between different organs in the body to control blood volume, pressure and osmolality, which are clearly closely related. The major hormones involved are arginine vasopressin (AVP), atrial natriuretic peptide (ANP) and aldosterone. AVP, also known as antidiuretic hormone (ADH), is secreted from the posterior pituitary and increases water resorption from urine. ANP is a hormone secreted by the right cardiac atrium that acts on the kidney to promote diuresis, with the loss of both water and sodium. Aldosterone is a mineralocorticoid secreted by the adrenal gland that increases sodium resorption in the kidney. Adrenaline and angiotensin II maintain blood pressure by acting directly on the blood vessels to produce constriction. BP, blood pressure.

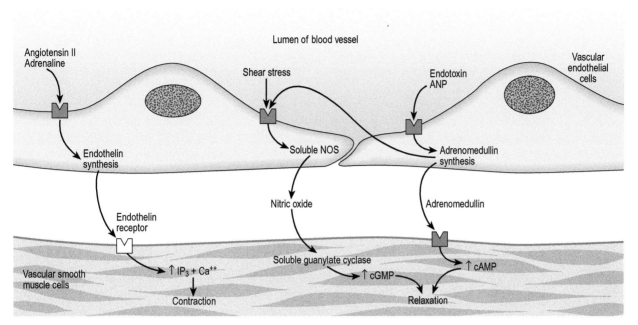

Figure 13.7 Paracrine regulation of local vascular tone. Vascular endothelial cells secrete a range of mediators in response to hormonal and other stimuli. These mediators include nitric oxide, endothelin and adrenomedullin. ANP, atrial natriuretic peptide; cGMP/cAMP, cyclic guanosine/adenosine monophosphate; IP$_3$, inositol triphosphate; NOS, nitric oxide synthase.

For example, in MEN1 it is more common to find all four parathyroid glands affected than just one.

As the MENs are inherited in an autosomal dominant manner, first-degree relatives of individuals with MEN may undergo genetic screening, with regular medical screening offered to those found to be carrying a *MEN* gene (Table 13.2). In the families of people with MEN2, specific screening for the *RET* proto-oncogene is carried out. This gene encodes a version of tyrosine kinase and so mutations are associated with disordered cell signalling and cell growth. Specific mutations in this gene are associated with a particularly aggressive form of medullary thyroid carcinoma at an early age. A thyroidectomy is performed in children found to be carrying the most significant mutations. This can be performed as early as 6 months of age.

Autoimmune polyglandular endocrinopathy

This is a rare group of diseases, characterized by the failure of more than one endocrine organ. The commonest form, type II, is also known as Schmidt's syndrome. It affects women more frequently than men and is associated with particular HLA genotypes. The glands most frequently affected are the adrenals, thyroid and endocrine pancreas.

Regulation of blood pressure and volume

The regulation of blood pressure and volume is achieved through the integration of many different hormonal and paracrine signals. Some of these mechanisms are shown

in Figure 13.6. The actions of aldosterone, angiotensin II and adrenaline are covered in detail in Chapters 5 and 6, and arginine vasopressin is considered in Chapter 3. The other hormone involved is atrial natriuretic peptide (ANP), a hormone secreted by the cells of the heart. This peptide acts on the kidney, via single-transmembrane ANP receptors (see Ch. 2), coupled to cyclic guanosine monophosphate (cGMP) signalling, to promote water and sodium loss in the urine. Figure 13.6 shows a simplified scheme of the major mechanisms involved in the systemic regulation of blood pressure.

In addition to the systemic regulation of blood pressure, there are several other factors that act at a local level to maintain local vascular tone (Fig. 13.7). There is evidence that nitric oxide secretion may be impaired in some patients with endocrine hypertension. It has also been suggested that adrenomedullin has a role in the vasodilatation associated with septic shock.

The next 100 years of endocrinology

We started this book by observing that endocrinology is a young scientific discipline, with 2005 being recognized as the centenary of its origin. Given the wealth of knowledge that has accumulated over the last 100 years, it is tempting to speculate what an edition of this book might contain in 2105. For the centenary edition of *The Endocrinologist*, the newsletter of The Society for Endocrinology, prominent scientists and clinicians working in the field were asked to predict the status of endocrinology in 100 years' time. One of the common themes to emerge was that our understanding of the detailed

MISCELLANEOUS HORMONES

interaction between different endocrine systems would be considerably greater by 2105. This 'integrated physiology', with an understanding of complex functions such as regulation of appetite, sexuality, reproduction, ageing and even body shape, could lead to tailoring of lifestyles by hormonal 'treatments'. Taken to its extreme, this argument suggests that we may even be able to use hormones to alter social behaviour. If these speculations turn out to be only partly true, it is clear that the next 100 years of hormone research will throw up many moral and ethical questions.

AII – angiotensin II.

AAS – anabolic androgenic steroids.

ABP – androgen binding protein, found in the testes.

ACE – angiotensin converting enzyme.

ACTH – adrenocorticotropic hormone, 5 corticotropin.

ADH – anti-diuretic hormone (AVP).

AME – apparent mineralocorticoid excess.

AMH – anti-müllerian hormone.

Androgens – the family of male sex steroids, including testosterone and androstenedione.

ANP – atrial natriuretic peptide.

aquaporin 2 – a protein on the apical membrane of cells lining the renal collecting ducts whose production is stimulated by AVP. This protein functions as a water channel.

autocrine – when the hormone acts locally, on the same type of cell that produces it.

AVP – arginine vasopressin.

bioassay – a method for measuring hormones based on the biological response they produce.

BMI – body mass index, calculated by: weight (kg)/ height squared (metres).

Bromocriptine – a dopamine agonist used to treat hyperprolactinaemia.

cAMP – cyclic adenosine monophosphate (a second messenger).

CBG – cortisol binding globulin (transcortin).

CCK – cholecystokinin.

cGMP – cyclic guanosine monophosphate.

climacteric – the period of time, which includes the menopause, when a woman's menstrual cycle becomes irregular and ceases, as a result of age.

COX – cyclooxygenase, enzymes involved in prostaglandin synthesis.

C-peptide – the connecting peptide, which is cleaved from the A- and B-peptides comprising mature insulin, and released into the circulation with insulin.

CRH – corticotropin releasing hormone.

CT – computed tomography, a scanning X-ray that can build up a two-dimensional slice picture or, with software, a three-dimensional image.

Cushing's disease – a condition of glucocorticoid excess caused by ACTH secretion from a pituitary tumour.

Cushing's syndrome – the symptoms of glucocorticoid excess, due to any cause, including the use of corticosteroids as a medicine.

CYP – a gene family that encodes the cytochrome P450 hydroxylase enzymes involved in steroid biosynthesis.

DAG – diacylglycerol.

DBP – vitamin D binding protein.

desmopressin – synthetic analogue of arginine vasopressin that can be administered orally or by nasal spray.

DHEA(S) – dehydroepiandrosterone (sulphate), the most abundant androgen secreted by the adrenal cortex.

DHT – 5a-dihydrotestosterone.

diurnal variation – the predictable daily pattern of secretion of a hormone.

dynamic test – the measurement of a hormone in response to an agent that normally either stimulates or suppresses its secretion.

ectopic hormone secretion – the inappropriate secretion of a hormone by a tissue that does not usually produce it.

EGF – epidermal growth factor.

endocrine – secretion of hormones directly into the bloodstream by a ductless tissue.

EPO – erythropoietin.

exocrine – secretion of the product of a gland via a secretory duct.

FFAs – free fatty acids.

FSH – follicle stimulating hormone.

GFR – glomerular filtration rate.

GH – growth hormone.

GHRH – growth hormone releasing hormone.

glucocorticoid – a class of steroid produced by the adrenal cortex that binds to the intracellular glucocorticoid (cortisol) receptor and has a role in the regulation of metabolism.

GLUT – a family of glucose transporter proteins.

GnRH – gonadotropin releasing hormone.

G protein – guanyl nucleotide binding protein.

HbA$_{1c}$ – glycated haemoglobin, a measure of 'average' blood glucose concentration.

hCG – human chorionic gonadotropin.

HDL – high-density lipoprotein.

HLA **gene** – human leucocyte antigen, a histocompatability locus gene.

Hormone – a chemical messenger that circulates in blood and acts by binding to specific receptors.

HPA axis – hypothalamo – pituitary–adrenal axis.

hPL – human placental lactogen.

HRE – hormone response element. An area in the promoter region of a gene that allows hormones to stimulate or repress gene transcription.

HRT – hormone replacement therapy.

hsp – heat shock proteins (associated with steroid receptors in the resting state).

hydrocortisone – the name given to cortisol when it is used therapeutically.

IDDM – type 1 diabetes mellitus (insulin-dependent diabetes mellitus).

IGF – insulin-like growth factor.

IP$_3$ – inositol trisphosphate, a second messenger.

IRS –insulin receptor substrate.

JAK–STAT – Janus-associated kinase–signal transducer and activator of transcription.

kinase – an enzyme that catalyses the phosphorylation of a substrate protein.

LDL – low-density lipoprotein.

LH – luteinizing hormone.

MAPK – mitogen-activated protein kinase.

MEN – multiple endocrine neoplasia.

menarche – a girl's first menstrual period.

menopause – permanent cessation of menstruation, defined as 12 months since the last monthly period.

mineralocorticoid – a class of steroid hormones secreted by the adrenal cortex that has a role in the regulation of salt balance.

mitosis – cell division.

MRI – magnetic resonance imaging.

NIDDM – type 2 diabetes mellitus (non-insulin-dependent diabetes mellitus).

NOS – nitric oxide synthase.

NSAIDs – non-steroidal anti-inflammatory drugs.

OGTT – oral glucose tolerance test.

osmolality – the number of osmoles per kilogram of solvent.

osmolarity – the number of osmoles per litre of solvent.

paracrine – when a hormone acts locally, within the same tissue, on a cell type that is different to the cell that secreted the hormone.

PCOS – polycystic ovarian syndrome.

PIP$_2$ – phosphatidylinositol bisphosphate.

PLA2 – phospholipase A2. An enzyme that converts membrane phospholipids to arachidonic acid; the first step in prostaglandin production.

plasma – whole blood that is prevented from clotting prior to centrifugation. Does not contain cells but does contain clotting factors.

PLC – phospholipase C. An enzyme involved in second messenger production.

PNMT – phenylethanolamine *n*-methyltransferase, the enzyme that catalyses the formation of adrenaline from noradrenaline.

polydipsia – excessive drinking (usually refers to non-alcoholic drinks).

polyuria – the production of excessive quantities of urine.

POMC – pro-opio-melanocortin.

portal system – a vascular connection with two sets of capillary beds.

PRL (Prl) – prolactin.

PTH – parathyroid hormone.

PTHrp – parathyroid hormone-related peptide.

reverse T3 – thyroxine that has had one iodine residue removed, producing an inactive hormone.

serum – the liquid component of blood without the cells, obtained by allowing whole blood to clot, then centrifuging the clot (including cells) away from the serum.

SHBG – sex hormone binding globulin.

SIADH – syndrome of inappropriate anti-diuretic hormone.

SRY – sex-determining region Y (testis determining factor).

StAR – steroidogenic acute regulatory protein.

T$_3$ – thyroxine that has had one iodine residue removed, producing an active hormone.

T$_4$ – thyroxine, thyroid hormone.

TeBG – testosterone binding globulin 5 SHBG.

TGFb – transforming growth factor b.

THBG – thyroid hormone binding globulin.

thyrotoxicosis – the clinical disease state caused by excess thyroid hormone.

TK – tyrosine kinase.

TRH – thyrotropin releasing hormone.

tropic hormones – hormones that regulate other endocrine glands.

TSH – thyroid stimulating hormone 5 thyrotropin.

VIP – vasoactive intestinal polypeptide.

Index